PREVENTION, TREATMENT AND REHABILITATION OF CARDIOVASCULAR DISEASE IN SOUTH ASIANS

EDITORS
Kiran C R Patel
Ajay M Shah

South Asian Health Foundation

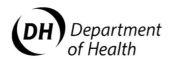

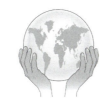

South Asian Health Foundation

LONDON: TSO

Published by TSO (The Stationery Office) and available from:

Online
www.tso.co.uk/bookshop

Mail, Telephone, Fax & E-mail
TSO
PO Box 29, Norwich, NR3 1GN
Telephone orders/General enquiries: 0870 600 5522
Fax orders: 0870 600 5533
E-mail: book.orders@tso.co.uk
Textphone 0870 240 3701

TSO Shops
123 Kingsway, London, WC2B 6PQ
020 7242 6393 Fax 020 7242 6394
68-69 Bull Street, Birmingham B4 6AD
0121 236 9696 Fax 0121 236 9699
9-21 Princess Street, Manchester M60 8AS
0161 834 7201 Fax 0161 833 0634
16 Arthur Street, Belfast BT1 4GD
028 9023 8451 Fax 028 9023 5401
18-19 High Street, Cardiff CF10 1PT
029 2039 5548 Fax 029 2038 4347
71 Lothian Road, Edinburgh EH3 9AZ
0870 606 5566 Fax 0870 606 5588

TSO Accredited Agents
(see Yellow Pages)

and through good booksellers

SAHF 2005

A CIP catalogue record for this book is available from the British Library

A Library of Congress CIP catalogue record has been applied for

First published 2005

ISBN 0 11 703608 0

Printed in the United Kingdom for The Stationery Office

Contents

List of Contributors

AH Barnett
Professor of Medicine and Consultant Physician, University of Birmingham and Heart of England NHS Foundation Trust, Birmingham

S Bellary
University of Birmingham and Heart of England NHS Foundation Trust, Birmingham

RS Bhopal
Bruce and John Usher Professor of Public Health, Community Health Sciences, College of Medicine and Veterinary Medicine, University of Edinburgh, Edinburgh, and Patron, South Asian Health Foundation

R Boyle
National Clinical Director for Heart Disease, Department of Health

FP Cappuccio
Clinical Sciences Research Institute, Warwick Medical School, UHCW Campus, Coventry

A Dixon
University of Birmingham and Heart of England NHS Foundation Trust, Birmingham

L Donaldson
Chief Medical Officer, Department of Health

S Gupta
Consultant Cardiologist, Department of Cardiology, Whipps Cross and St Bartholomew's Hospitals, London

MP Kelly
Director of Research, Health Development Agency, London

S Korn
Imperial College School of Medicine, Hammersmith Hospital, London

R Leslie
Clinical Physiotherapy Specialist for Cardiac Rehabilitation Services,
New Cross Hospital, Wolverhampton

G Mathews
Project Co-ordinator, Khush Dil, Edinburgh

KCR Patel
Consultant Cardiologist, Sandwell and West Birmingham Hospitals NHS Trust,
West Bromwich, Honorary Senior Lecturer in Cardiovascular Medicine,
University of Birmingham and Chair of Trustees, South Asian Health Foundation

N Patel
Life Peer, House of Lords and Patron, South Asian Health Foundation

M Rawlins
Director, National Institute for Clinical Excellence, London

N Sahni
Coronary Heart Disease Asian Link Nurse, New Cross Hospital, Wolverhampton

AM Shah
British Heart Foundation Professor of Cardiology, King's College London School of
Medicine at Guy's, King's College and St Thomas' Hospitals, London, and Patron,
South Asian Health Foundation

P Sharma
Imperial College School of Medicine, Hammersmith Hospital, London

P Weissberg
Medical Director, British Heart Foundation

Q Zaidi
British Heart Foundation, London

Foreword

The epidemic of coronary heart disease has been and continues to be a significant challenge in the UK. South Asian communities, those with birth or ancestral origins in the Indian subcontinent, are a vital part of the social and economic fabric of modern, multicultural Britain. It is no surprise that for South Asians, exposure to a new environment and a new way of life has exposed health issues which are different from those in their countries of origin. Second and third generation South Asians are also showing patterns of disease which differ to their white European counterparts. Coronary heart disease is an important example of such health issues, and was the subject of a conference addressing prevention, treatment and management strategies in South Asians. Coronary heart disease remains one of the leading killers in our country. Exploring the reasons for its even greater impact in South Asian communities living in Britain is an important area for research. Assessing the evidence to enable an effective public health response to treatment and rehabilitation strategies is a major challenge. The SAHF conference brought together a truly multidisciplinary field consisting of leading researchers, experts and healthcare professionals with practical experience in this field. They are all to be congratulated for the quality of their contributions and, more than this, for their commitment to finding solutions to the problem of coronary heart disease in the South Asian communities living in Britain.

This publication, based upon the proceedings of the conference, will bring this important issue to a much wider audience and, we believe, enable many others to come forward to help advance understanding of the problem and to take action to combat it.

Lord Naren Patel, Patron, The South Asian Health Foundation

Sir Liam Donaldson, Chief Medical Officer, Department of Health

Sir Michael Rawlins, National Institute for Health and Clinical Excellence

Professor Peter Weissberg, British Heart Foundation

Preface

Coronary heart disease (CHD) poses a massive challenge globally. The last 50 years have witnessed an explosion of research from bench to bedside to population to explore the multifactorial aetiology of CHD. There is significant heterogeneity in the risk of CHD and it is now clear that populations of South Asian origin in the West have substantially greater relative CHD mortality and morbidity than the indigenous population. In December 2004, the South Asian Health Foundation (SAHF), with the support of the British Heart Foundation and the Department of Health, organised a UK symposium on the 'Prevention, Treatment and Rehabilitation of Cardiovascular Disease in South Asians: Implementing Good Practice'. The meeting brought together leading researchers and organisations active in the field of ethnicity and coronary disease in an attempt to galvanise efforts to tackle and manage this epidemic. This book summarises and updates the proceedings of the symposium, with the aim to disseminate this vital information. On behalf of the SAHF, we hope that this book will highlight important and relevant issues pertinent to the management of South Asian patients with CHD.

Kiran C R Patel

Ajay M Shah

Acknowledgements

We would like to thank the authors who have provided exceptional contributions to this book and, indeed, to the field of ethnicity and cardiovascular disease. Without their effort, progress in this field would be severely compromised. We also wish to thank the many individuals and bodies who have made this publication possible and acknowledge the efforts of the SAHF Patrons and Trustees. The British Heart Foundation and Department of Health have provided funding towards this publication, which enables us to distribute it widely. We also wish to thank Schering Plough for sponsoring delegates to the original symposium in 2004.

Responsibility

The editors accept responsibility for the compilation and editing of this volume on behalf of the South Asian Health Foundation. The final responsibility for the accuracy of the content, however, rests with the named authors of each chapter.

The South Asian Health Foundation

The South Asian Health Foundation was founded in 1999. It seeks to promote improvements in the quality of, and access to, health care and health promotion in South Asians; and to promote scholarship and research that lead to those objectives. Our work at a grass roots level includes community based meetings delivered throughout the UK. Our national membership aims to enable all South Asian communities, organisations and healthcare professionals to benefit equally and effectively from health promotion and education, thus building upon the good work which already exists in many regions and ensuring that all South Asian communities benefit from these efforts. In 2001, SAHF hosted a UK symposium on ethnicity and CHD: 'The Epidemic of Coronary Heart Disease in the South Asian populations: Causes and Consequences'. In 2004, SAHF hosted a conference: 'Prevention, Treatment and Rehabilitation of Cardiovascular Disease in South Asians: Implementing Good Practice'. The latter symposium has resulted in this book. SAHF is working closely with several organisations, including the Department of Health, the British Heart Foundation and the National Heart Forum, to facilitate achievement of its objectives.

For more information, contact SAHF at info@sahf.org.uk or Dr Kiran Patel, Chair of Trustees, SAHF, 39 Westfield Road, Edgbaston, Birmingham, West Midlands B15 3QE. www.sahf.org.uk

Glossary[1]

Glossary of terms relating to ethnicity and race used in this book

African: A person with African ancestral origins who self-identifies as African, but excluding South Asians.

Afro-Caribbean: A person of African ancestral origins whose family settled in the Caribbean before coming to Britain and who self-identifies as Afro-Caribbean. *See also Black.*

Bangladeshi: A person whose ancestry lies in the Indian subcontinent who self-identifies as Bangladeshi. *See also South Asian.*

Chinese: A person with ancestral origins in China, including Hong Kong, who self-identifies as Chinese.

Ethnicity: [a] The social group a person belongs to, and both identifies with and is identified with, as a result of a mix of cultural and other factors including language, diet, religion, ancestry, and race. *See also race.*

European: Effectively, this is a synonym for White *(see below)*.

Indian: A person whose ancestry lies in the Indian sub-continent who identifies as Indian. (NB: Major changes to India's geographical boundaries took place in 1947.) *See also South Asian.*

Pakistani: A person whose ancestry lies in the Indian subcontinent who identifies as Pakistani. *See also South Asian.*

Race: The group a person belongs to as a result of a mix of physical features (e.g. skin colour, hair texture), ancestry and geographical origins, as identified by others or, increasingly, as self-identified. The importance of social factors in the creation and perpetuation of racial categories has led to the concept broadening to include social and political heritage, making its usage similar to ethnicity. Race and ethnicity are increasingly used as synonyms. *See also ethnicity.*

South Asian: A person whose ancestry is in the countries of the Indian subcontinent, that is, India, Pakistan, Bangladesh and Sri Lanka. *See also, Indian, Pakistani, Bangladeshi.*

White: The term usually used to describe people with European ancestral origins who identify as white (sometimes called European, Caucasian or Caucasoid). The word is capitalised to highlight its specific use.

[a]   The concepts of race and ethnicity are so intertwined that consideration of one necessarily requires consideration of the other. In this proposal, the term ethnicity is used except when there is clear distinction between this and race.

Reference

1.   Bhopal RS. Glossary of terms relating to ethnicity and race: for reflection and debate. *Journal of Epidemiology and Community Health* 2004; **58**:441-445.

1
Coronary heart disease in South Asians: the scale of the problem and the challenges ahead

Sandeep Gupta

Introduction

Coronary heart disease (CHD) remains the leading cause of death in the United Kingdom (UK), accounting for around 300,000 deaths per year.[1] South Asians (i.e. those with ancestral origins on the Asian subcontinent) have a 40–50% greater mortality from CHD compared to the indigenous white European population.[1] Although the first published evidence of the excess CHD risk in South Asians came as early as 1959 from a study based on expatriate Indians in Singapore,[2] multiple subsequent studies from different countries have consistently highlighted this problem of premature CHD mortality. For the UK population, similar data have been available for at least 3 decades and mortality statistics have remained unchanged in this time.[3–5]

With the realisation of the burden of CHD in the UK in general and an imbalance in provision of cardiac services, the National Service Framework (NSF) in CHD was launched in 2000.[6] Some 5 years on, some successes include a reduction in waiting times for coronary angiography and subsequent revascularisation procedures, increased prescribing rates of secondary preventative agents in primary and secondary care, and a large number of Rapid Access Chest Pain Clinics, Heart Failure and Cardiac Rehabilitation services set up nationwide. In this short period since the launch of the NSF, the age-standardised mortality from CHD in the UK has fallen by 22%.[7] For South Asians, the excess burden of CHD remains but their plight is now receiving heightened awareness, with agencies such as the Department of Health (DoH), British Heart Foundation (BHF) and South Asian Health Foundation (SAHF) helping to address issues in a vigorous and concerted campaign.[8]

Why do South Asians have premature CHD mortality?

The answer to this question remains unclear but inevitably will be part genetic and part environmental. Several hypotheses have been generated. The most convincing attributes the excess CHD mortality to the higher prevalence of the metabolic syndrome (comprising insulin resistance, hypertension, central obesity and dyslipidaemia) and diabetes mellitus in South Asians. Insulin resistance in this population may appear as early as childhood and supports the concept (at least in part) of a genetic predisposition.[9, 10] The other proposed mechanisms include disadvantaged socio-economic status, a 'proatherogenic' diet and a relative lack of physical activity.[11] Furthermore, high levels of homocysteine and Lp(a), endothelial dysfunction, and inflammation are other possibilities.[11] However, none of the proposed hypotheses have been systematically evaluated with a prospectively designed population based (cohort) study. Most of the existing evidence on CHD in South Asians is derived from case control and cross-sectional studies with a particular scarcity of information on stroke. The findings of the recently published INTERHEART study suggest that more than 80% of the global burden of CHD, irrespective of country of origin, can be attributed to conventional cardiac risk factors.[12] This raises the question 'why are South Asians at such heightened risk?' It may be that certain risk factors have increased 'potency' in this population compared to white Europeans. Targets for optimal body mass index (BMI) are already lower in South Asians than white Europeans, and the question arises as to whether total cholesterol targets should also be set at lower ranges. If not potency alone, the interaction(s) among risk factors may be different in South Asians compared to other populations.

Comparing and contrasting South Asians

Emerging data highlights that South Asians are a heterogeneous group with respect to CHD risk. Bangladeshis fare the worst, followed by Pakistanis and then Indians.[13] Some of the disparity may be related to variation in the prevalence of risk factors such as smoking, poverty and socio-economic status amongst subgroups. Bangladeshis have greater unemployment rates, poorer uptake of childhood immunisations, more dental caries, etc. South Asians in general are more likely to present late to hospital following chest pain and less likely to be prescribed all of the available secondary prevention medications compared to white Europeans,[14] the reasons for this being unclear. Furthermore, South Asians are less likely to take up revascularisation procedures,[15] and more likely to decline and drop out from cardiac rehabilitation programmes.[8] All of these factors potentially contribute to a more adverse cardiovascular outcome. Of additional relevance is the presentation of CHD. South Asians are more likely to present with 'atypical' symptoms and more likely to be diagnosed as 'non-cardiac' despite having established CHD.[16] It can hence be comprehended how CHD in South Asians might go undetected and undiagnosed, and appropriate treatments delayed, if clinical history alone is used. It is imperative to increase awareness of ethnicity as a risk factor and the rudimentary requirement to use objective assessments should not be denied to these populations (e.g. ECG, exercise ECG, troponin, etc.).

Issues surrounding primary prevention in South Asians

It is suggested that health inequalities are further widening, with the CHD mortality rate in South Asians falling at a rate much lower than the rest of the population.[1] The first step towards addressing this disparity should target primary prevention of CHD. This may be achieved by targeted risk assessment and early lifestyle changes (such as smoking cessation, increased physical activity and increased consumption of fruits and vegetables) and/or pharmacological intervention (such as lipid-lowering medication) in the high-risk second and third generation South Asians. At the core of any prevention lies the concept of risk assessment. Unfortunately, a CHD risk estimation tool validated in this ethnic group is currently non-existent. The available scales such as the Framingham, FINRISK and the SCORE systems (derived from cohort studies of American and European white populations) have been shown to underestimate CHD risk in South Asians,[17] as Cappuccio will discuss in chapter 3. Furthermore, the 'normal' ranges for independent risk factors for CHD (such as blood pressure, body mass index [BMI] and lipid profile) derived from studies on western population may be too high for South Asians. It follows that intervention driven by these ranges may potentially result in undertreatment of the CHD risk in this population. Therefore, the threshold for intervention and goals for treatment should perhaps be set lower for South Asians by 10%–20%, compared to white Europeans, similar to recommendations for patients with diabetes mellitus. The hypothesis that all South Asians are 'pre-diabetic' may be an oversimplification but might help to make preventative targets and therapies easier to institute.

What has been achieved so far?

The DoH and the BHF (as Zaidi discusses in chapter 8) have played a key role in increasing the awareness of excess CHD burden among South Asians in the UK and various strategies and projects are now in fruition. The publication of the DoH document 'Heart Disease in South Asians' has aided to highlight Good Practices and community-based projects nationwide.[18] The BHF-funded production of written and visual information and other resources in key South Asian languages is novel and aims to enhance the communication of all aspects of heart disease for these communities. Specific campaigns targeting South Asian women (who have 50% greater death rates from CHD than white European women) have been delivered. Finally, the funding of several community and research projects (such as Project Dil in Leicester,[19] the CADISAP study in East London[20] and BRUM study in Birmingham[21]) has been critical in practically and scientifically addressing the issues of risk factors within differing South Asian groups. The recently formed SAHF is aiming to enhance the collaboration of all established agencies to define key areas of need in research, assessment, prevention and therapy, with a particular focus on cardiovascular disease.

A personal view: what could or should be done next?

An increase in awareness among public and health care professionals about the excess risk of CHD in South Asians is paramount. This would involve utilising literature and other resources, conferences and workshops, and specific consensus guidelines (now being considered), but also not underestimating the power and influence of the media, community link workers and organisations to educate the populations at risk.

The establishment of 'well-Asian clinics' to screen high-risk second and third generation South Asians for CHD followed by early appropriate pharmacological and lifestyle interventions (such as smoking cessation, increased consumption of fruits and vegetables, and increased physical activity) should be considered. Adopting lower thresholds and lower target-driven prevention strategies (similar to those used for patients with diabetes mellitus) may be a simplistic but very practical approach, but may require more robust scientific evidence, as Barnett et al discuss in chapter 6. Another key issue is to ensure that health services offered are culturally, religiously and linguistically appropriate for the varying South Asian groups, which will enhance the uptake and compliance of the population at risk. Finally, the importance of well designed large cohort studies to formally clarify the aetiological basis for the excess CHD risk in South Asians cannot be over-emphasized. Such research will inevitably be of relevance to South Asians settled not only in the UK, but also in other developed and developing countries (e.g. the Indian subcontinent) where CHD rates are ever-increasing.

The ensuing chapters will explore in more detail the various facets of the excess CHD risk in South Asians, and help to provide both a source of debate and inspiration on how further to enhance our knowledge and address the colossal task ahead.

References

1. Coronary heart disease statistics 2004: British Heart Foundation Statistics: website www.heartstats.org

2. Danaraj T, Acker M, Danaraj W, Ong W, Yam T. Ethnic group differences in coronary heart disease in Singapore: an analysis of necropsy records. *Am Heart J* 1959; **58**: 516–526.

3. McKeigue P, Sevak L. *Coronary heart disease in South Asian communities*. London: Health Education Authority, 1994.

4. Bhatnagar D, Anand I, Durrington P, Patel D, Wander G, Mackness M, et al. Coronary risk factors in people from the Indian subcontinent living in west London and their siblings in India. *Lancet* 1995; **345**: 405–409.

5. Gupta S, Belder A, and Hughes L. Avoiding premature coronary deaths in Asians in Britain. *Br Med J* 1995; **311**: 1035–1036.

6. Department of Health National Service Framework for Coronary Heart Disease: March 2000.

7. Department of Health National Service Framework for Coronary Heart Disease: Progress report 2004.

8. Kuppuswamy V, Gupta S. Excess Coronary Deaths in South Asians in UK: Problem highlighted but more to be done. *Br Med J* 2005; **330**: 1223–4.

9. Whincup P, Gilg J, Papacosta O, Seymour C, Miller G, Alberti K, Cook D. Early evidence of ethnic differences in cardiovascular risk: cross sectional comparison of British South Asian and white children. *Br Med J* 2002; **324**: 635.

10. Saxena S, Ambler G, Cole T, Majeed A. Ethnic group differences in overweight and obese children and young people in England: Cross sectional survey. *Archives of Disease in Childhood* 2004; **89**:30–6.

11. Patel K and Bhopal S. *The epidemic of coronary heart disease in South Asian populations: causes and consequences.* 2004. Chapters 2–7.

12. Yusuf S, Hawken S and Ounpuu S. Effects of potentially modifiable risk factors associated with myocardial infarction in 52 countries (the INTERHEART study): case-control study. *Lancet* 2004; **364**: 937–52 .

13. Bhopal R, Unwin N and White M. Heterogeneity of coronary heart disease risk factors in Indian, Pakistani, Bangladeshi, and European origin populations: cross sectional study. *Br Med J* 1999; **319**: 215–220.

14. Ward P, Noyce P, St Leger A. Multivariate regression analysis of associations between general practitioner prescribing rates for coronary heart disease drugs and healthcare needs indicators. *J Epidemiol Community Health* 2005; **59**: 86.

15. Feder G**,** Crook A, and Magee P. Ethnic differences in invasive management of coronary disease: prospective cohort study of patients undergoing angiography. *Br Med J* 2002; **324**: 511 – 516.

16. Barakat K, Wells Z, Ramdhany S, Mills P, Timmis A. Bangladeshi patients present with non-classic features of acute myocardial infarction and are treated less aggressively in east London, UK. *Heart* 2003; **89**: 276–9.

17. Bhopal R, Fischbacher C, Vartiainen E, Unwin N, White M, Alberti G. Predicted and observed cardiovascular disease in South Asians: application of FINRISK, Framingham and SCORE models to Newcastle Heart Project data. *Journal of Public Health* 2005; **27**: 93–100.

18. Department of Health. Heart disease and South Asians: Delivering the National Service Framework for Coronary Heart Disease. Best Practice Guideline 2004.

19. Farooqi A, Bhavsar M. Project Dil: a co-ordinated Primary Care and Community Health Promotion Programme for reducing risk factors of coronary heart disease amongst the South Asian community of Leicester – experiences and evaluation of the project. *Ethnicity Health* 2001; **6**: 265–70.

20. Kuppuswamy V, Jhuree J, and Gupta S. Coronary Artery Disease In South Asian Prevention (CADISAP) Study: a culturally sensitive cardiac rehabilitation (CR): can it improve uptake and adherence of CR among South Asians? *Heart* 2004; **90** (suppl II: abstract 177; A51).

21. Jolly K, Lip GY, Sandercock J. Home-based versus hospital-based cardiac rehabilitation after myocardial infarction or revascularisation: design and rationale of the Birmingham rehabilitation uptake maximisation study (BRUM): a randomised controlled trial. *BMC Cardiovasc Disord* 2003; **3**: 10.

2
The challenge of changing patient behaviour

Michael P Kelly

Introduction

Much ill health has, at least in part, its origins in human behaviour. Many cancers, heart disease and a number of other illnesses such as obesity, type 2 diabetes, HIV and chlamydia are, to an important degree, the outcome of the way we behave and the way we live. Smoking, eating too much fatty food, not consuming enough fresh fruit and vegetables and not taking enough exercise, all contribute significantly to the risk of disease. None of these behaviours are involuntary, but are, at least theoretically, within the realms of individual choice and responsibility. However, given the prevalence of heart disease, cancer, diabetes, obesity, sexually transmitted infections and so on in the population, many people clearly do not exercise those choices in ways that are beneficial to their health.

It is important, therefore, to consider the role of health behaviour and the possibility of behaviour change as a means of preventing these illnesses. Over the years at different times, various governments and local agencies have tried to get people in the population at large to change their behaviour in health-enhancing ways.[1, 2] The campaigning activities of organisations such as the Health Education Council, the Health Education Authority, the Health Education Board for Scotland and the Health Development Agency were based on the principle of health gain following from behaviour change.[3] Certainly, a huge dividend of prevention is within grasp if only people would, or could, change their behaviour![4, 5]

There are many different types of interventions which may be deployed to help to change behaviour. They vary from those which aim to increase knowledge and awareness of services to help to prevent risk, to interventions which seek to change attitudes and motivations, for example by communicating messages about the harm that smoking does to the lungs and cardiovascular system. Another of the methods typically employed focuses on increasing physical or interpersonal skills, for example on how to use condoms, or how to use assertiveness skills in sexual encounters. Some interventions are designed to change beliefs and perceptions, like those aimed at increasing testicular self-examination in men by raising their awareness of risk and normalizing self-examination. Another approach is to influence social norms, for example about public perceptions of the harm of second-hand smoke inhalation, or public acceptance of breast feeding.

Among South Asian populations in Britain, the diseases which cause the greatest amounts of morbidity and mortality include those in which individual behaviour plays an important role. South Asians have higher mortality rates from and are more likely to die prematurely from coronary heart disease (CHD) than the general population, as described by Gupta in chapter 1. These disparities are worsening.[6] While many factors are implicated in the aetiology of these diseases, the role of behaviour is an element that requires attention. This chapter considers what the current literature has to offer; there are two main strands in the literature, one psychological and one sociological.

The psychological approach

Underlying the efforts to bring about behaviour change is a considerable body of scientific psychological literature.[7–9] The original impetus for this research occurred when the first effective vaccines against poliomyelitis were manufactured.[10] The problem psychologists sought to understand was the following: notwithstanding the availability of an effective vaccine, its uptake was relatively low. In fact, there was an epidemic of cases of polio in the USA *after* the development and availability of the vaccine. Two questions therefore emerged. What were the factors that led to this type of resistant behaviour? And what could be done to change it? The answers came to be explained by what was called the Health Belief Model.[11, 12] Models which have been designed to answer these sorts of questions have since applied to many different health behaviours such as the use of contraception, smoking cessation, oral health, taking exercise and alcohol misuse.[9]

The health belief model[11, 12] describes a logical process of conscious decision making, whereby behaviour change occurs in response to perceived vulnerability to harm and to cue stimuli. People, it is suggested, have a *lay* sense of the extent to which they are susceptible to a particular health problem. They also have in their minds a sense of how serious the disease is. These, so the model argues, feed into a kind of cognitive calculus in which is also included a *lay* estimate of the degree of threat posed by the disease. Then, factored into their mental equation or estimate of risk is, once again, a *lay assessment* of the benefits of and the barriers to doing something to protect from or prevent the disease. This then predicts the likelihood of taking preventive or health promoting action. Stimuli might include mass media campaigns or the experience of a frightening health event such as chest pain.

Historically, users of this model have focused on simple rather than complex behaviours, for example getting an injection rather than negotiating safer sex. It is important to note that lay assessments of susceptibility, severity and threat are precisely that, they are *lay* beliefs. They do not correspond to medical assessments of the problem nor its seriousness. It is also important to note that originally at any rate, the model focused on well-defined medical conditions rather than more general health problems or concerns. Lay people's assessment of risk will be subject to all kinds of factors located in their background and education, friendship networks and the way they relate to media about medical matters. It is also important to note that lay people do not necessarily think in terms of well-defined disease categories. Their thoughts about their health, depending on the individual, will likely be much more diffuse.

Another influential model is the stages of change model or trans-theoretical model.[13, 14] This conceives of behaviour change as a process, with different factors intervening at each step. People's readiness and willingness to change is viewed as a process of increasing readiness. The stages are defined as: pre-contemplation; contemplation; preparation; action; maintenance; termination. The change processes are not viewed as irreversible or unidirectional. The stages of change models emphasize the need to know where the targeted population is in terms of stage, then to deliver the stage-matched intervention. The model is premised on the notion that people move through similar stages of change as a consequence of therapeutic interventions regardless of the intervention being applied. Moreover, there is an orderly sequence of change, although some people move more rapidly than others and some seem to get stuck at particular stages for periods of time. The implication of this model is that different interventional approaches are required at different stages of the change process. This model has been heavily used in health promotion in, for example, smoking cessation, alcohol use, exercise and screening.[14–16]

A third important approach is the theory of planned behaviour (TPB). This is based on an earlier model called the theory of reasoned action;[17] this theory emphasizes behavioural intentions as the outcome of a combination of several beliefs. It is applied to aspects of human behaviour that are under conscious control.[18] The TPB suggests that behavioural intention is the key determinant of behaviour. This is influenced by three components. These are a person's attitude towards undertaking the behaviour, the perceived social pressure to adopt the behaviour (the subjective norm), and perceived behavioural control. The TPB addresses perceptions of control with outcomes strongly correlated with behavioural intention. Behavioural intentions are considered to be an outcome of attitudes towards a behaviour (such as immunisation), subjective norms (social values, peer pressure and individuals' perceptions of whether these norms apply to them), and perceived behavioural controls (how much control an individual feels they have over their behaviour).

It is also worth noting the information-motivation-behavioural skills model.[19, 20] This directly links to the skill deficits which people have when trying to change behaviour. Behavioural skills are described as both an objective ability and perceived self-efficacy. The skills may be technical or personal.

There are many other models. What is interesting is that reviews of the effectiveness of interventions[21] have found that interventions using a theory- or model-based approach to behaviour change – regardless of which theory or model was used – tended to be more effective than those that did not, indicating perhaps that using a theory-based approach to plan interventions may make an intervention better planned and delivered. Models provide the basis for increased rigour in intervention design. Model-based interventions are necessarily more explicit. Exner et al[22] identify an important design component as 'having explicitly stated goals or hypotheses, with clearly operationalized outcomes'. Models require that the intervention articulates the determinants that influence behavioural and clinical outcomes and are explicit about which of these they propose to change; how they propose to change them; how they will demonstrate that change; and how if at all that change has contributed to a behavioural or clinical outcome.

There are a number of general points to make about psychological models. They help us to know why as well as whether an intervention is effective, shedding light on the extent to which elements of interventions can be applied in different contexts with different populations. Different models work better in relation to some conditions or preventive actions rather than others. Approaches that can accommodate irrational behaviour and incorporate the function of wider determinants tend to cover a broader range of potential issues, but to be less good when dealing with specifics and guiding interventions. No single theory or model has universal applicability and the choice of a particular approach should depend on what the focus for change is. No single theory or model can universally predict behavioural intentions or outcomes for all populations, although many can accurately predict and describe some changes particularly when they are focused on the individual. They tend to be less good at incorporating structural or socioeconomic factors.

Models tend to operate at fairly high levels of generality. This obviously aids simplification and understanding. On the other hand it can make applying them to real-world situations a little tricky because real life tends to be complex and messy. Models which are multi-level, i.e. which operate at the individual *and* social level and which take into account the needs and the characteristics of particular population groups, work best. Unfortunately the more particular the local characteristics and needs of the population are, the more complex models become, and the advantages of simplicity can get lost. So in real-life interventions, practitioners change and amend models to suit their needs. While this of course is an entirely sensible thing to do from a practical point of view, it often means that the models do not appear to work very well from a scientific point of view.

There are however two scientific limitations associated with these types of models – empirical and theoretical. The empirical problem is that where the models are used there is sometimes considerable variance in their predictive power. Unfortunately, it is not very easy to tell whether this is caused by poor design and method or underlying weakness in the models. However, given the propensity for practitioners to change components of the model to suit their needs, what we really have in the evidence is a vast array of the results of testing of slightly different models. The reason for this is the need to ground the models in the real world and to operationalize the components in them to suit local circumstances. It is also very important to acknowledge that notions such as attitude, intention, belief and assessment of risk are much easier to talk about in the abstract than to apply to real settings and to real people.

The theoretical problem is more serious. This is about the explanatory focus on the individual to the exclusion of the social level of explanation in these models and many like them. Where social factors are included in these models, they are invariably treated as characteristics of individuals and hence as part of an individually driven explanation, rather than explanatory causes in their own right. Consequently, social structure is not dealt with adequately. It is treated as a set of individually expressed factors, not as a highly variegated pattern of social arrangements requiring their own level of analysis, irreducible to the individual. The population is not homogeneous. It is heterogenous and its component parts respond to the same interventions in different ways. However, these models generally assume universal precepts about human behaviour or treat social differences as confounding factors in the analysis. In other words the key differences between social classes, men and women, ethnic groups, young and old and residential circumstances are treated as background or contextual factors, rather than important determining factors in their own right. Different segments of the population respond in very different ways to the same intervention by virtue of their social differences, and attempting to apply general principles across the whole population tends to underemphasise the important role of social difference.[23, 24]

The other very significant problem with this body of work is the degree to which it pays scant attention to specific population groups such as South Asians. There are a few studies published which deal with the health belief model applied to these groups,[25, 26] but the literature is dominated by American studies.[27–29] Some studies have called into serious question the validity of such models across different population groups especially the theory of planned behaviour[30] whereas others have suggested that the trans-theoretical model is robust across different population groups.[27, 31] The fact is these models have not been applied in any systematic way to ethnically diverse populations[32] and this is especially marked in the context of the UK South Asian population. Given the popularity of these models and the extent to which they have been widely used as the basis for all sorts of interventions, this is a serious gap in the literature.

In spite of the general problems attaching to these approaches, it is important to remember that from a practical point of view, the logical imperfections and scientific limitations of these models are much less important than their ability to help us to bring about change in real time for real people. These models help to direct and provide us with a framework for thinking about interventions. If they are treated as a recipe for determining exactly what should be done, in each and every circumstance, they will disappoint. If they are treated as signposts for action, they can be very helpful indeed.[33] In the context of the South Asian population the potentials of these models are yet to be realised.

Sociological approaches

At about the same time as psychologists began to construct models to understand behaviour change, American sociologists, building on a much older tradition in the medical literature,[34–37] began to investigate the different ways in which people access and make use of services and to develop models to explain these behaviours by using social and cultural (rather than individual) factors. The starting point was the work of David Mechanic on help seeking.[38–40] Mechanic noted that modern medicine was very effective for alleviating pain and suffering. However, the population seemed to behave in non-rational ways in terms of its pattern of use of and access to services. The questions being explored were: why don't people act rationally in the face of illness, and why don't they seek immediate medical help when there is something wrong with them? The answers lay in the social worlds in which people lived. The research showed that pathways to treatment were frequently tortuous and that delay, especially in the most serious conditions like cancer, was very common.[41] To complicate matters still further, there were also lots of people who misused the services available and consulted inappropriately, using up valuable and scarce practitioner time for apparently trivial complaints.[42]

There are a large number of models that can be drawn upon here.[41,43,44] The broad thrust of these models highlights a number of factors, but at the heart of them is a notion of the importance of culture and belief. These cultural patterns and beliefs are in turn related to the position of groups and individuals in the social structure. In other words, not only is people's behaviour in the face of illness complex and grounded in the context of their everyday lives, their ability to change habitual ways of thinking and acting about health and illness is also deeply engrained and consequently difficult to change.

The main arguments to emerge from this considerable literature are:

- That individuals engage in complicated self-assessments of their own health, the seriousness of their symptoms, and their estimation of the likelihood that medical science will be able to help, prior to their taking action.

- These assessments are closely linked to the degree of threat which the individual imagines attaches to their symptoms.

- Their responses are culturally and socially patterned along the lines of locality, ethnicity, class and gender. Assessment of symptoms and evaluations of threat are linked to the social worlds people inhabit.

- There can be important and highly localised triggers to taking action.

- Information in and of itself is part of the solution, but is heavily mediated via lay understandings and lay information.

- Once a decision has been made to seek help the person may well follow a route to self-medication or alternative therapy, as well as and/or instead of a route to mainstream medical services.

- Cultural and social networks play an important mediating role and, for some groups, the role of lay experts of various kinds has been demonstrated to be important.

So in summary, patterns of behaviour in the face of illness, and when making decisions about alleviating threat or doing something which will reduce risk, are based on a very complex set of costs and benefits on the part of the person affected. Attitudes play a very significant role, but behaviours are overlaid by cultural and social factors, and routes to the doctor and decisions to take a health-enhancing action are frequently lengthy and convoluted. However, behaviours can be plotted and patterns identified within certain fairly well-defined parameters. The most important message that this literature conveys is that the way people make use of services and take preventive actions is not universal even when the provision of service is universal. Patterns of response are highly varied and therefore any intervention designed to change, moderate or mediate in some way the way people use services will have to be highly differentiated and tailored to the needs of particular population groups. In other words, services need to be culturally and socially sensitive.

This type of sociologically oriented approach has been applied to South Asian populations in the UK, and it offers an important potential line of research and development. The research has focused on a range of well-defined issues and problems which help to contextualise the health of South Asians. So topics like professional–patient communications,[45] help-seeking behaviour,[46–49] and barriers to access[50–52] have all been explored. There has been extensive work done on health beliefs within this particular cultural milieu.[53–59] Gradually, therefore, a very rich picture is emerging of the cultural factors which impact on the health of South Asians and other groups. However, what is missing so far is a systematic way of linking this knowledge and understanding to the delivery of services, to the interface of people and the professions.

Conclusion

This brief consideration of the literature has demonstrated a number of points. First, health-related behaviour may have an important role to play in the prevention of those diseases which are significant causes of mortality and morbidity in the South Asian population (and of course many other groups). Second, there is a rich psychological literature which offers some well-tested approaches to behaviour change, which although open to scientific criticism, offers a reasonable way forward. Third, the principal models used in health behaviour change have not been tested extensively with sub-populations in Britain (although the picture is a little better in North America), and therefore the transferability of the knowledge remains to be demonstrated. Fourth, there is very deep and emerging sociological and sociologically-informed literature on the ways that cultural milieux impact on health behaviour and therefore potentially provide clues to preventive activities. Finally, these clues have not yet been applied at all extensively either to the provision of services or to the processes of change which will help to reduce the significant burden of premature mortality and morbidity in the South Asian population.

References

1. Department of Health and Social Security (1976). *Prevention and Health: Everybody's Business*. London: HMSO.

2. Killoran A, Fentem P, Caspersen C (1994). *Moving On: International Perspectives on Promoting Physical Activity*. London: Health Education Authority.

3. Health Development Agency, (2002). *Cancer Prevention: A resource to support local action in delivering the NHS Cancer Plan*. London: Health Development Agency.

4. Kelly MP and Capewell S (2004). *Relative contributions of changes in risk factors and treatment to the reduction of coronary heart disease mortality*. London: Health Development Agency.

5. Kelly MP, Crombie H, Owen L (2004a). *The contribution of smoking, diet, screening and treatment to cancer mortality in the under 75s*. London: Health Development Agency.

6. Fox C (2004). *Heart Disease and South Asians: Delivering the National Service Framework for Coronary Heart Disease*. London: Department of Health.

7. Halpern D, Bates C, Beales G, Heathfield A (2003). Personal responsibility and behaviour change. Cabinet Office Strategic Audit paper. London: Strategy Unit.

8. Ho R, Davidson G, Ghea V. Motives for the adoption of protective health behaviours for men and women: an evaluation of the psychosocial-appraisal health model. *Journal of Health Psychology* 2005; **10**: 373–95.

9. Kaplan RM, Sallis JF and Patterson TL (1993). *Health and Human Behavior*. New York: McGraw Hill.

10. Levine AJ (1992). *Viruses.* New York: Scientific American Library.

11. Rosenstock IM (1974). Historical origins of the health belief model. *Health Education Monograph* 2: 328–335.

12. Rosenstock IM. Social learning theory and the health belief model. *Health Education Quarterly* 1988; **15**(**2**): 175–183.

13. Prochaska JO and DiClemente CC (1992). Stages of change in the modification of problem behaviors. In: Herson M, Eisler R and Miller PM (eds), *Progress in Behavior Modification.* Sycamore, IL: Sycamore Publishing: 183–218.

14. DiClemente CC, Prochaska JO, Fairhurst SK, Velicer WF, Velasquez MM, and Rossi JS. The process of smoking cessation: an analysis of pre-contemplation, contemplation, and preparation stages of change. *Journal of Consulting and Clinical Psychology* 1991; **59**: 295–304.

15. Riemsma RP, Pattenden J, Bridle C et al (2002). A systematic review of the effectiveness of interventions based on a stages-of-change approach to promote individual behaviour change. *Health Technology Assessment* 6 (24).

16. Riemsma RP, Pattenden J, Bridle C et al. Systematic review of the effectiveness of stage based interventions to promote smoking cessation. *British Medical Journal* 2003; **326**: 1175–1177.

17. Fishbein M and Azjen I (1975). *Belief, Attitude, Intention and Behavior: An Introduction to Theory and Research*. Reading MA: Addison-Wesley.

18. Azjen I (1985). From intentions to actions: a theory of planned behaviour. In: Kuhl J and Beckman J (eds). *Action Control from Cognition to Behaviour*. New York: Springer-Verlag: 11–39.

19. Fisher JD and Fisher WA (2000). Theoretical approaches to individual-level change in HIV risk behaviour. In: Peterson JL and Di Clemente RJ. *Handbook of HIV Prevention*. New York: Kluwer Academic/Plenum Publishers.

20. Fisher WA and Fisher JD (2003). A general social psychological model for changing AIDS risk behavior. In: Pryor J and Reeder G (eds). *The Social Psychology of HIV Infection*. Hillsdale, NJ: Erlbaum: 127–153.

21. Roe L, Hunt P, Bradshaw H et al. (1997). *Health Promotion Effectiveness Reviews 6: Health Promotion Interventions to Promote Healthy Eating in the General Population*: a review. London: Health Education Authority.

22. Exner TM, Seal DW and Ehrhardt AA. A review of HIV interventions for at-risk women. *AIDS and Behavior* 1997; **1**: 93–124

23. Killoran A and Kelly MP. Towards an evidence-based approach to tackling health inequalities: the English experience. *Health Education Journal* 2004; **63**: 7–14.

24. Graham H and Kelly MP (2004) *Health inequalities: concepts, frameworks and policy*. London: Health Development Agency.

25. McAllister G and Farquhar M. Health beliefs: a cultural division? *Journal of Advanced Nursing* 1992; **17**: 1447–54.

26. Ahmad F, Cameron JI, Stewart DE. A tailored intervention to promote breast cancer screening among South Asian immigrant women. *Social Science and Medicine* 2005; **60**: 575–586.

27. Davits SL, Fish L and Kohler CL. Transtheoretical model of change among hospitalized African American smokers. *American Journal of Health Behavior* 2004: 145–150.

28. Godin G, Matickatyndale E, Adrien A, Mansonsinger S, Willms D, Cappon P. Cross-cultural testing of three social cognitive theories – an application to condom use. *Journal of Applied Social Psychology* 1996; **26**: 1556–1586.

29. Hamm RM, Juniper KC, Kerby DS, Oman RF. The relationships among constructs in the Health Belief Model and the Transtheoretical Model among African-American college women for physical activity. *American Journal of Health Promotion* 2004; 354–357.

30. Trost SG, Pate RR, Dowda M, Ward DS, Felton G, Saunders R. Psychosocial correlates of physical activity in white and African-American girls. *Journal of Adolescent Health* 2002; 226–233.

31. Rodgers WM, Courneya KS, Bayduza AL. Examination of the transtheoretical model and exercise in 3 populations, *American Journal of Health Behavior* 2001; 25: 33–41.

32. Adams TB, Hallion ME, Pagell F, Spencer L. Applying a transtheoretical model to tobacco cessation and prevention: a review of literature. *American Journal of Health Promotion* 2002; 7–71.

33. Kelly MP, Speller V, Meyrick J (2004). *Getting evidence into practice in public health.* London: Health Development Agency.

34. Cobb B. Why do people detour to quacks? *The Psychiatric Bulletin* 1954a; **3**: 66–9.

35. Cobb B, Clarke RL, McGuire C, Howe CD. Patient responsible delay of treatment in cancer: a social psychological study. *Cancer* 1954b; **7**: 920–26.

36. Cobb S, Bauer W, Whiting I. Environmental factors in rheumatoid arthritis: a study of the relationship between the onset and exacerbation of arthritis and the emotional or environmental factors, *Journal of the American Medical Association* 1939; **113**: 668–670.

37. Apple D. How laymen define illness. *Journal of Health and Human Behaviour* 1960; **1**: 219–25.

38. Mechanic D. The concept of illness behaviour. *Journal of Chronic Disease* 1962; **15**:189–94.

39. Mechanic D (1972). Response factors in illness: the study of illness behaviour, in Jaco, EG (ed). *Patients, Physicians and Illness: A Sourcebook in Behavioural Science and Health*, 2nd ed. New York: Free Press.

40. Mechanic D and Volkart EH. Illness behaviour and medical diagnosis. *Journal of Health and Human Behavior* 1960; **1**: 86–94.

41. Anderson R (1988). The development of the concept of health behaviour and its application to recent research. In: Anderson R, Davies JK, Kickbusch I, McQueen DV and Turner J. *Health Behaviour Research and Health Promotion*. Oxford: Oxford University Press.

42. Millward LM and Kelly MP (2004). Doctors' perceptions of their patients. In: Jones R, Britten N, Culpepper L, Gass DA, Grol R, Mant D and Silagy C (eds). *Oxford Textbook of Primary Medical Care.* Oxford: Oxford University Press; 181–185.

43. Dingwall R (1976). *Aspect of Illness.* London: Martin Robertson.

44. Albrecht G (ed) (1994). *Advances in Medical Sociology: A Reconsideration of Health Behavior Change Models.* London JAI Press.

45. Ahmad WI, Kernohan EE, Baker MR. Patients' choice of general practitioner: influence of patients' fluency in English and the ethnicity and sex of the doctor. *Journal of the Royal College of General Practitioners* 1989; **39**:153–5.

46. Ahmad WI, Kernohan EE, Baker MR. Patients' choice of general practitioner: importance of patients' and doctors' sex and ethnicity. *British Journal of General Practice.* 1991a ; **41**: 330–1.

47. Ahmad WI, Baker MR, Kernohan EE. General practitioners' perceptions of Asian and non-Asian patients. *Family Practice* 1991b; **8**: 52–6.

48. Bhugra D and Hicks MH. Effect of an educational pamphlet on help-seeking attitudes for depression among British South Asian women. *Psychiatric Services* 2004; **55**: 827–9.

49. Joshi MS (1998). Adherence in ethnic minorities: the case of South Asians in Britain. In: Myers LB and Midence K (eds). *Adherence to Treatment in Medical Conditions.* Amsterdam, Netherlands: Harwood Academic Publishers.

50. Chapple A. Vaginal thrush: perceptions and experiences of women of south Asian descent. *Health Education Research* 2001; **16**: 9–19.

51. Gatrad AR and Sheikh A. Palliative care for Muslims and issues before death. *International Journal of Palliative Nursing* 2002; **8**: 526–31.

52. Hawthorne K. Asian diabetics attending a British hospital clinic: a pilot study to evaluate their care. *British Journal of General Practice* 1990; **40**: 243–7.

53. Bhopal RJ. The interrelationship of folk, traditional and western medicine within an Asian community in Britain. *Social Science and Medicine* 1986; **22**: 99–105.

54. Bhopal RJ. Bhye bhaddi: a food and health concept of Punjabi Asians. *Social Science and Medicine* 1986; **23**: 687–8.

55. Bush HM, Williams RG, Lean ME, Anderson AS. Body image and weight consciousness among South Asian, Italian and general population women in Britain. *Appetite* 2001; **37**: 207–15.

56. Dein S. Explanatory models of and attitudes towards cancer in different cultures. *Lancet Oncology* 2004; **5**:119–24.

57. Horne R, Graupner L, Frost S, Weinman J, Wright SM, Hankins, M. Medicine in a multi-cultural society: the effect of cultural background on beliefs about medications. *Social Science and Medicine* 2004; **59**:1307–13.

58. Lip GY, Khan H, Bhatnagar A, Brahmabhatt N, Crook P, Davies MK. Ethnic differences in patient perceptions of heart failure and treatment: the West Birmingham heart failure project. *Heart* 2004; **90**: 1016–9.

59. Farooqi A, Nagra D, Edgar T and Khunti, K. Attitudes to lifestyle risk factors for coronary heart disease amongst South Asians in Leicester: a focus group study. *Family Practice* 2000; **17**: 293–297.

3
Predicting risk and its role in prescribing

Francesco P Cappuccio

Introduction

Cardiovascular disease is the most common and yet one of the most preventable causes of death in the western world. The unprecedented economic development in Asia and the rapid urbanisation of Africa are associated with rapid changes in lifestyle and environmental exposures, so that the burden of chronic cardiovascular diseases is rising rapidly in developing countries.[1] The risk of premature cardiovascular disease (CVD) varies by ethnic group. Relative to white subjects, people of African origin, both Caribbeans and West Africans, have a high incidence of stroke and end-stage renal failure, whereas coronary heart disease (CHD) is less common.[2-4] On the other hand, South Asians from the Indian subcontinent and East Africa have a much higher incidence of CHD,[2-4] as discussed by Gupta in chapter 1. Further examination of the mortality from CHD in South Asian populations overseas indicates that this higher risk appears to be a feature of these populations across the world, whether recently migrated or not.[4] This is also true when the reference host population is at different risk, such as in England where it is high, or in the Singaporean Chinese where it is low. Similarly, the mortality from stroke in African-Americans is high, whether born in the United States or in the Caribbean.[4,5] It is also important to note that mortality and morbidity from end-stage renal disease varies by ethnic group, with a much greater burden in both people of African origin and of people from the Indian subcontinent living in the United Kingdom.[6]

In this review, we will pay particular attention to the commonest traditional risk factors present in ethnic minority populations living in the UK, which are likely to account for a large proportion of the CVD they experience. However, throughout the review we will highlight aspects that require further attention.

Hypertension

There is consensus that, amongst people of African origin, hypertension is three to four fold more prevalent than in the white European UK population.[7,8] This is true for men and women and is present at any age, at least in adulthood. This observation fits with the excess risk of stroke and renal disease in these populations.[3,9] African-Americans also show an increase in the prevalence and severity of hypertension,[10] as do Caribbeans[10,11] and urban black African populations.[10] Hypertension has also been associated with all-cause mortality in rural Africa[12] and with vascular and renal complications.[13]

The prevalence of hypertension appears to be significantly higher in some studies of South Asian immigrants in the UK compared to Europeans[7,8,14] and in both rural and urban populations living in India.[15,16] This contrasts with some reports both in the UK and in the South Asian groups living in Tanzania.[17,18] The high prevalence of hypertension in certain South Asian groups and in people of African origin, particularly in view of their low smoking rates, is likely to contribute to the high mortality from stroke experienced by these groups in the UK.[2,3]

Detection, management and control of hypertension

Such high prevalence rates and subsequent complications raise the issue of how to reduce this burden of hypertension. There is evidence to suggest that the 'rule of halves' by which only a small proportion of people with hypertension receive appropriate management and adequate control, has improved over the years.[19] People of black African origin in the UK are more likely to have their hypertension detected in the community when compared to other ethnic groups.[7] This may indicate greater awareness amongst patients and doctors of the importance of controlling hypertension in black populations. However, observations of the level of adequacy of management reveal that these black populations tend not to achieve good blood pressure control.[7] This may be due to several factors e.g. more severe hypertension, inadequate drug therapy due to individual sensitivity to different drugs, lack of concordance with therapy, specific doctors' beliefs, organisational pitfalls, etc. It is now established that the quality of hypertension control predicts mortality from stroke. Furthermore, stroke-related events in people with known hypertension but with inadequate blood pressure control can be regarded as unacceptable and avoidable events.[20] Therefore the need for improvement of community-based care of hypertension is of paramount importance in programmes for the prevention of stroke, particularly in the elderly and in black populations.

The first step for the prevention and management of hypertension is non-pharmacological.[21] Lifestyle and dietary modifications should be implemented. For hypertension, it is particularly important to aim at a reduction of sodium intake to about 50–80 mmol/day (equivalent to 3–5g of daily salt intake). This is most useful in the populations of African origin who are particularly sensitive to the detrimental effect of high salt intake and, for the same reason, respond best to a reduction in sodium intake.[22] Reduction in sodium intake and an adequate potassium intake by increasing the amount of fruit and vegetable consumption should, for instance, be considered for the prevention of hypertension and stroke particularly in communities of black African origin both in the UK and also in developing countries of Africa where urbanisation is associated with an increase in salt intake, a reduction in potassium intake, and more sedentary lifestyle and an increase in body weight. Likewise, control of body weight should be emphasised in overweight women of black African origin.

British hypertension guidelines suggest that people with severe hypertension (blood pressure consistently $\geq$160/100 mmHg) or those with mild-to-moderate hypertension (blood pressure consistently between 140–159/90–99 mmHg) and either diabetes, target organ damage or cardiovascular complications should be treated.[23] However, in the 1999 version of the guidelines, in those with mild-to-moderate hypertension without diabetes, target organ damage or cardiovascular complications, the decision to treat was made on the basis of a 10-year CHD risk estimate (taken from the Framingham equations) $\geq$15% (assumed to be equivalent to a 10-year CVD risk >20%). Whilst the latter equivalence holds in white populations, it does not for ethnic minority populations, since CHD risk underestimates CVD risk. Indeed, the use of a 10-year risk of CHD $\geq$15% to decide how to manage people with mild-to-moderate uncomplicated hypertension would identify for treatment of 91% of white people but only 81% of South Asians and people of African origin (Figure 3.1).[24] If we used a lower threshold for the CHD risk (for example, 12% and 10%) in South Asians and in people of African origin with mild-to-moderate uncomplicated hypertension, we would have a higher probability of identifying and treating those with a 10-year CVD risk ≥20% (Figure 3.1).[24] However, the use of the CVD risk would be an even better measurement.[25] Two recent studies have compared predicted CHD risk with that expected by mortality rates in South Asians. One of them found discrepancies between predicted risks by ethnic groups and standardised mortality ratio by country of birth.[26] The other found that a Framingham score and the FINRISK score both gave expected predictions, but the SCORE model did not.[27] It is important to note that both the FINRISK[27] and the SCORE[28] models only use mortality, therefore assuming a constant case-fatality rate across ethnic groups. The overall CVD risk is based on both morbidity and mortality (i.e. incidence of disease). Finally, one study examined the sensitivity and specificity of different strategies for adjusting the Framingham score for South Asians, and found that adding 10 years to the age provided the simplest way of making Framingham risk match an assumed excess risk of 1.79 in South Asian people.[29] Ideally, a calibration of the Framingham score using prospective data, as carried out in American ethnic groups,[30] would be needed. Unfortunately, prospective studies in ethnic minority groups in the UK are lacking. Pending further evidence, the latest BHS-IV guidelines have taken a pragmatic approach and have amended the criteria recommending now the use of the Framingham score. The latest BHS-IV guidelines have amended the criteria, recommending now the use of CVD risk as a guide to hypertension

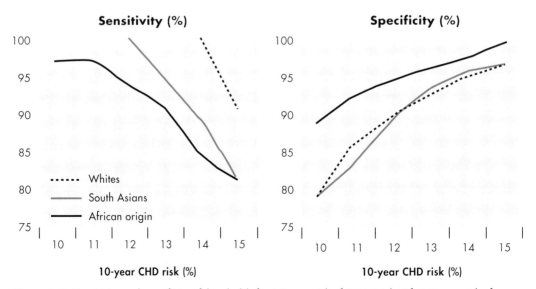

Figure 3.1 Sensitivity and specificity of thresholds for 10-year risk of CHD to identify 10-year risk of CVD ≥20% in different ethnic groups after exclusion of people with diabetes, target organ damage and cardiovascular complications. (ADAPTED FROM CAPPUCCIO ET AL 2002[24])

management in the mild-to-moderate group to avoid inequalities across hypertensive patients of different ethnic background.[31]

Once non-pharmacological treatment has failed to reduce blood pressure to within target ranges (currently $\leq$140/85 mmHg and $\leq$140/80 mmHg in diabetics),[23] then pharmacological treatment is required. The general strategies for the management of hypertension with monotherapy and with combination therapy have been recently highlighted by the British Hypertension Society.[23, 26, 32] In particular, for patients over the age of 55 years or those of black African origin, guidelines recommend initial monotherapy with either a calcium channel blocker or a thiazide diuretic.[32] If blood pressure is not controlled, combination therapy should be considered with the addition of either an angiotensin converting enzyme inhibitor (ACEI) or an angiotensin receptor blocker (ARB) to the original monotherapy. Less preferred, but nevertheless acceptable, would be the addition of a beta-blocker. If the blood pressure were still not controlled, then step three would be the combination with a thiazide diuretic, a calcium channel blocker and either an ACEI or an ARB. All these would be implemented on the background of non-pharmacological management, which would be based mainly on a reduction in daily sodium intake to less than 80 mmol and a control of body weight in overweight or obese individuals.

Type 2 diabetes

The prevalence of type 2 diabetes is far higher in urban South Asians than white Europeans.[7, 33] This is true either when using the WHO definition of diabetes (based on the results of an Oral Glucose Tolerance Test) or the more contemporary definition of the American Diabetic Association (based on fasting serum glucose only). However, it should be noted that the new fasting ADA diagnostic criteria of diabetes give a markedly lower prevalence than the new full WHO criteria, including post glucose load levels.[34] Furthermore the ADA criteria fail to identify subjects with impaired glucose tolerance, more prevalent amongst South Asians.[34]

The excess of diabetes in South Asians is remarkably constant in surveys of South Asian populations overseas, even when migration occurred many generations earlier.[4] This suggests that genetic factors may be important in determining susceptibility to diabetes.

Furthermore, recent evidence suggests that the very early signs of type 2 diabetes, such as hyperinsulinemia and central adiposity, are already present very early in life.[35] People of African origin also display a higher prevalence of type 2 diabetes when compared to European whites.[7, 36] More detailed metabolic studies, along with population-based investigations, have consistently identified a pattern of inter-correlated metabolic disturbances to be associated with type 2 diabetes in South Asian populations. These are hyperinsulinaemia, raised triglycerides and low HDL cholesterol levels, central adiposity with a high waist circumference and a high waist-to-hip ratio, altogether indicating a condition of insulin resistance and contributing to the metabolic syndrome.[7, 36] In contrast to this pattern, in people of African origin, type 2 diabetes is associated with a metabolic pattern that, despite the presence of raised glucose intolerance and high insulin levels, does show low triglycerides and high HDL cholesterol levels, a different distribution of adiposity with body mass index being a better measure of obesity particularly in black women.[7, 36] It is of interest that the outcome of patients with type 2 diabetes of African-Caribbean origin is not worse than that of white European diabetics.[37] In particular, African-Caribbean diabetics retain the lower levels of CHD mortality of their white counterparts when compared to South Asians. This suggests very strongly that there must be protective factors that play an important role. Besides the low triglycerides and high HDL-cholesterol, likely contributors could be the tendency to lower plasma homocysteine[38] and fibrinogen levels[39] and the lower level of adhesion molecules such as ICAM-1, VCAM-1 and P-selectin.[40]

In a survey in South London, white European people with diabetes were less likely to have been diagnosed than the other ethnic groups.[7] This suggests that the greater awareness of a higher prevalence of diabetes among ethnic minorities has led to a greater detection rate by primary care teams. An alternative explanation could be the accelerated progression of diabetes in these ethnic groups, leading to more symptoms and higher rates of diagnosis. Although this may be true for South Asians, it is not the case for those of African origin. It is surprising, therefore, that the treatment of diabetes was more common among people of African origin, although diabetes is not more aggressive in this ethnic group. One reason for the greater detection in black Africans could be the close association between hypertension and diabetes. Patients with hypertension are more likely to have diabetes and, conversely, patients with diabetes have a greater chance of having hypertension.

Management of hypertension in type 2 diabetics

Hypertension is very common in type 2 diabetes. It is strongly related to obesity and central adiposity and is highly predictive of cardiovascular and microvascular complications. Data from the UKPDS study[41] and from the HOT study[42] strongly support the view that anti-hypertensive treatment is more effective than glycaemic control in the prevention of micro- and macro-vascular disease as well as survival in type 2 diabetics. Furthermore, a tighter blood pressure control (to a lower threshold than non-diabetics) is associated with further cardiovascular protection. Therefore, recent guidelines recommend lowering blood pressure in hypertensive diabetics below 130/80 mmHg.[26]

Metabolic syndrome

This syndrome has become increasingly common. It is characterised by a clustering of metabolic risk factors in one individual. The metabolic syndrome is closely linked with a generalised metabolic disorder called 'insulin resistance' in which tissue responsiveness to the normal action of insulin is impaired. Specific definitions vary (Table 3.1), but essentially, the syndrome is characterised by abdominal adiposity, atherogenic dyslipidaemia, raised blood pressure, insulin resistance and/or glucose intolerance, and a prothrombotic and proinflammatory state. This syndrome is believed to accentuate the risk of CHD at any given

Table 3.1 Definitions of the metabolic syndrome (M (male), F (female), BMI (body mass index), DM (Type 2 diabetes mellitus), IGT (impaired glucose tolerance), FPG (fasting plasma glucose), TG (triglyceride), HDL (high density lipoprotein), LL (lipid lowering))

	World Health Organisation 1999	European Group of Insulin Resistance 1999	NCEP ATP III 2001	IDF 2005
	DM/IGT/ Ins Rest + 2 of following	Ins Rest + 2 of following	3 or more of following	Waist criteria + 2 others (FPG>5.6 or DM)
BMI (Kg/m²) Waist:Hip ratio	BMI>30 or W:H >0.9 (M) or > 0.85 (F)	Waist >94cm (M), >80(F)	Waist >102cm (M), >88cm (F)	Waist >94cm (M) or 80cm (F)
Dyslipidaemia (mM)	TG>1.7 or HDL <0.9(M),<1.0(F)	TG>2.0 or HDL<1.0	HDL<1.0(M). <1.3(F)	TG>1.7 or on LL therapy HDL<1 (M) or <1.2(F)
Hypertension (mmHg)	>140/90	>140/90	>135/85	>130/85 or on Rx
	Microalbuminuria			

level of LDL cholesterol. Recently the Adult Treatment Panel III[43] in the US has suggested a clinical definition of metabolic syndrome as the presence of three or more risk factors. Impaired fasting glucose usually is an indicator of insulin resistance and is frequently associated with other metabolic risk factors. A proportion of people with impaired fasting glucose will eventually develop type 2 diabetes, with further risk of developing CHD. Type 2 diabetes is, therefore, considered the epitome of the metabolic syndrome.

The prevalence of the metabolic syndrome varies substantially by ethnic groups.[44] However, whilst it is more frequent amongst South Asian Hindus as well as Muslims, it is not greatly raised in people of black African origin (both Caribbeans and West Africans). This is mainly due to the different pattern of dyslipidaemia, with South Asians displaying an atherogenic profile (high triglycerides and low HDL-cholesterol) and the black African people showing a more 'protective' atherogenic profile (low triglycerides and high HDL-cholesterol). However, the prevalence of diabetes and hypertension is much greater amongst people with the metabolic syndrome, with the expected gradient across ethnic groups.[44]

Other factors

A variety of other factors are thought to explain some of the ethnic differences in cardiovascular risk (Table 3.2). Recent evidence of a tendency to lower plasma fibrinogen[39] and homocysteine,[38] higher vitamin C[45] and lower levels of some circulating adhesion molecules in people of black African origin[40] supports the view that a cluster of protective factors might in part explain the reduced risk of CHD in African populations. At the same time, additional risk factors such as increased homocysteine,[38] small LDL particles,[46] raised PAI-1[47] and sialic acid[48] may help to explain the increased risk of CHD in South Asians. For instance, plasma homocysteine is raised only in South Asian Hindus, but not in Muslims, whereas it tends to be low amongst black Africans[38] (Figure 3.2). When adjusting for vegetarianism, the differences amongst Hindus were grossly attenuated, though not abolished. This suggests that cultural practices amongst vegetarian Hindus, such as the prolonged cooking of vegetables that destroys up to 90% of folate content, may be directly responsible for these findings. Indirect support is provided by the lower levels of plasma vitamin C (heat-labile vitamin) found amongst

Table 3.2 Differences in risk factors for cardiovascular disease in South Asians and people of black African origin living in the UK compared to whites

Factor (Reference)	South Asians	People of black African origin
Blood Pressure [8, 14, 36]	High (in Hindus and Muslims)	Very high
Body mass index [36]	–	Very high (in women)
Waist-to-Hip ratio [36]	Very high	Very high (in women)
Total serum cholesterol [36]	–	–
Serum triglycerides [36]	Very high	Low
Serum HDL-cholesterol [36]	Low	High
Serum insulin [36]	Very high	High
Serum glucose [36]	Very high	High
Hypertension [7, 8]	High	Very high
Diabetes [7]	Very high	High
Obesity [7]	High	Very high
Metabolic syndrome	Very high	High
Smoking [7, 14]	Low	Low
Alcohol intake [14]	–	Low
Physical activity [55]	Low	
Plasma fibrinogen [39, 47]	–	Low
Plasma vitamin C [45]	Low	–
Plasma homocysteine [38, 56]	High (in Hindus)	Low
Small Dense LDL [46]	High	
PAI-1 activity [47]	High	
Factor VII:C [47]	Low	
ICAM-1 [40]	–	Low
VCAM-1 [40]	–	Low
P-selectin [40]	–	Low
Lipid hydroperoxide [57]		High
Serum sialic acid [48]	High	–
Microalbuminuria [58,59]	High	High

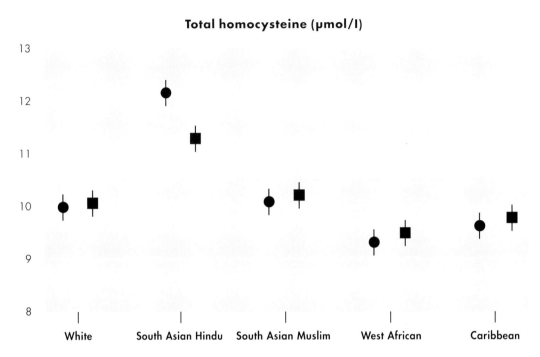

Figure 3.2 Plasma fasting total homocysteine levels (geometric mean and 95% CI) in people from different ethnic sub-groups, aged 40–59 years, living in South London, after adjustment for age, sex, body mass index and smoking (model 1 as circles) and after further adjustment for vegetarianism (model 2 as squares). P<0.001 by analysis of co-variance. BASED ON CAPPUCCIO ET AL[38]

South Asians.[45] Likewise, the lower levels in blacks could be consistent with more fruit and raw vegetables consumed as part of their diet.

Genetic factors

Both hypertension and diabetes have high heritability and run in families. It is therefore likely that both are under important genetic influences, probably due to several genes. The discussion of the genetics of hypertension and diabetes is beyond the scope of this review. However, great interest is given to possible gene-gene and gene-environment interactions (the adaptation-dysadaptation hypothesis) to help explain ethnic differences in cardiovascular risk. An example is the study of gene polymorphisms with implications for hypertension in black African populations,[49–52] for lipoprotein metabolism,[53,54] fibrinogen[39] and for homocysteine levels.[38]

References

1. Ezzati M, Lopez AD, Rodgers A, Vander Hoorn S, Murray CJL. Selected major risk factors and global and regional burden of disease. *Lancet* 2002; **360**:1347–60.

2. Balarajan R. Ethnic differences in mortality from ischaemic heart disease and cerebrovascular disease in England and Wales. *Br Med J* 1991; **302**: 560–4.

3. Wild S, McKeigue P. Cross sectional analysis of mortality by country of birth in England and Wales, 1970–92. *Br Med J* 1997; **314**: 705–10.

4. Cappuccio FP. Ethnicity and cardiovascular risk: variations in people of African ancestry and South Asian origin. *J Hum Hypert* 1997; **11**: 571–6.

5. Fang J, Madhavan S, Alderman MH. The association between birthplace and mortality from cardiovascular causes among black and white residents of New York City. *N Engl J Med* 1996; **335**:1545–51.

6. Raleigh VS. Diabetes and hypertension in Britain's ethnic minorities: implications for the future of renal services. *Br Med J* 2001; **314**: 209–13.

7. Cappuccio FP, Cook DG, Atkinson RW, Strazzullo P. Prevalence, detection and management of cardiovascular risk factors in different ethnic groups in South London. *Heart* 1997; **78**: 555–63.

8. Primatesta P, Bost L, Poulter NR. Blood pressure levels and hypertension status among ethnic groups in England. *J Hum Hypert* 2000; **14**: 143–8.

9. Raleigh VS, Kiri V, Balarajan R. Variations in mortality from diabetes mellitus, hypertension and renal disease in England and Wales by country of birth. *Health Trends* 1996; **28**: 122–7.

10. Cooper RS, Rotimi C, Ataman S, McGee D, Osotomehin B, Kadiri S et al. The prevalence of hypertension in seven populations of West African origin. *Am J Public Health* 1997; **87**: 160–8.

11. Poulter NR, Cappuccio FP, Chaturvedi N, Cruickshank JK. High blood pressure and the African-Caribbean community in the UK. Birmingham: MediNews Ltd, 1997.

12. Kaufman JS, Rotimi CN, Brieger WR, Oladokum MA, Kadiri S, Osotomehin BO et al. The mortality risk associated with hypertension: preliminary results of a prospective study in rural Nigeria. *J Hum Hypert*. 1996; **10**: 461–4.

13. Plange-Rhule J, Phillips R, Acheampong JW, Saggar-Malik AK, Cappuccio FP, Eastwood JB. Hypertension and renal failure in Kumasi, Ghana. *J Hum Hypert* 1999; **13**: 37–40.

14. Whitty CJ, Brunner EJ, Shipley MJ, Hemingway H, Marmot MG. Differences in biological risk factors for cardiovascular disease between three ethnic groups in the Whitehall II study. *Atherosclerosis* 1999; **142**: 279–86.

15. Gupta R, al Odat NA, Gupta VP. Hypertension epidemiology in India: meta-analysis of 50 year prevalence rates and blood pressure trends. *J Hum Hypert*. 1996; **10**: 465–72.

16. Gupta R, Sharma AK. Prevalence of hypertension and subtypes in an Indian rural population: clinical and electrocardiographic correlates. *J Hum Hypert* . 1994; **8**: 823–9.

17. Agyemang C, Bhopal RS. Is the blood pressure of South Asian adults in the UK higher or lower than that in European white adults? A review of cross-sectional data. *J Hum Hypert* 2002; **16**: 739–51.

18. Ramaiya KL, Swai AB, McLarty DG, Bhopal RS, Alberti KGMM. Prevalences of diabetes and cardiovascular disease risk factors in Hindu Indian subcommunities in Tanzania. *Br Med J* 1991; **303**: 271–6.

19. Primatesta P, Brookes M, Poulter NR. Improved hypertension management and control. Results from the Health Survey for England 1998. *Hypertension* 2001; **38**: 827–32.

20. Du X, Cruickshank JK, McNamee R, Saraee M, Sourbutts J, Summers A et al. Case-control study of stroke and the quality of hypertension control in Northwest England. *Br Med J* 1997; **314**: 272–6.

21. Cappuccio FP, Siani A. Non-pharmacologic treatment of hypertension. In: Crawford MH, Di MArco JP eds. *International Textbook of Cardiology. Section 3: Hypertensive Heart Disease*, p 7.1–7.10. London-Edinburgh-New York-Philadelphia-St Louis-Sydney-Toronto: Mosby International 2001.

22. He FJ, Markandu ND, Sagnella GA, MacGregor GA. Importance of the renin system in determining blood pressure fall with salt restriction in black and white hypertensives. *Hypertension* 1998; **32**: 820–4.

23. Ramsay LE, Williams B, Johnston GD, MacGregor GA, Poston L, Potter JF et al. Guidelines for management of hypertension: report of the third working party of the British Hypertension Society. *J Hum Hypert* 1999; **13**: 569–92.

24. Cappuccio FP, Oakeshott P, Strazzullo P, Kerry SM. Application of Framingham risk estimates to ethnic minorities in the UK and implications for primary prevention in general practice: a cross-sectional population based study. *Br Med J* 2002; **325**: 1271–4.

25. Gomez GB, Kerry SM, Oakeshott P, Rowlands G, Cappuccio FP. Changing from CHD to CVD risk-based guidelines for the management of mild uncomplicated hypertension in different ethnic groups: implications for primary care. *J Hum Hypert* 2005; **19**: 321–4.

26. Quirke TP, Gill PS, Mant JW, Allan TF. The applicability of the Framingham coronary heart disease prediction function to black and minority ethnic groups in the UK. *Heart* 2003; **89**: 785–6.

27. Bhopal R, Fischbaker C, Vartiainen E et al. Predicted and observed cardiovascular disease in South Asians: application of FINRISK, Framingham and SCORE models to Newcastle Heart Project data. *J Public Health* 2005; **27**: 93–100.

28. Conroy RM, Pyorala K, Fitzgerald AP et al. Estimation of ten-year risk of fatal cardiovascular disease in Europe: the SCORE project. *Eur Heart J* 2002; **24**: 987–1003.

29. Aarabi M, Jackson PR. Predicting coronary risk in UK South Asians: an adjustment method for Framingham-based tool. *Eur J Cardiovasc Prev Rehabil* 2005; **12**: 46–51.

30. D'Agostino RB sn, Grundy S, Sullivan LM et al. Validation of the Framingham coronary heart disease prediction scores: results of a multiple ethnic groups investigation *JAMA* 2001; **286**: 180–7.

31. Williams B, Poulter NR, Brown MJ et al. Guidelines for management of hypertension: report of the fourth working party of the British Hypertension Society, 2004 – BHS IV. *J Hum Hypert* 2004; **18**: 139–85.

32. Brown MJ, Cruickshank JK, Dominiczak AF, MacGregor GA, Poulter NR, Russell GI et al. Better blood pressure control: how to combine drugs. *J Hum Hypert* 2003; **17**:81–6.

33. McKeigue PM, Shah B, Marmot MG. Relation of central obesity and insulin resistance with high diabetes prevalence and cardiovascular risk in South Asians. *Lancet* 1991; **337**: 382–6.

34 Harris TJ, Cook DG, Wicks PD, Cappuccio FP. Impact of the new American Diabetes Association diagnostic criteria for diabetes and impaired fasting glucose on subjects from three different ethnic groups living in the UK. *Nutr Metab Cardiovasc Dis* 2000; **10**: 305–9.

35. Whincup PH, Gilg JA, Papacosta O, Seymour C, Miller GJ, Alberti KGMM et al. Early evidence of ethnic differences in cardiovascular risk: cross sectional comparison of British South Asian and white children. *Br Med J* 2002; **324**: 625–6.

36. Cappuccio FP, Cook DG, Atkinson RW, Wicks PD. The Wandsworth Heart & Stroke Study. A population-based survey of cardiovascular risk factors in different ethnic groups. Methods and baseline findings. *Nutr Metab Cardiovasc Dis* 1998; **8**: 371–85.

37. Chaturvedi N, Jarrett J, Morrish N, Keen H, Fuller JH. Differences in mortality and morbidity in African Caribbean and European people with non-insulin dependent diabetes mellitus: results of 20 year follow up of a London cohort of a multinational study. *Br Med J* 1996; **313**: 848–52.

38. Cappuccio FP, Bell R, Perry IJ, Gilg J, Ueland PM, Refsum H et al. Homocysteine levels in men and women of different ethnic and cultural background living in England. *Atherosclerosis* 2002; **164**: 95–102.

39. Cook DG, Cappuccio FP, Atkinson RW, Wicks PD, Chitolie A, Nakandakare ER et al. Ethnic differences in fibrinogen levels: the role of environmental factors and the b-fibrinogen gene. *Am J Epidemiol* 2001; **153**: 799–806.

40. Miller MA, Sagnella GA, Kerry SM, Strazzullo P, Cook DG, Cappuccio FP. Ethnic differences in circulating adhesion molecules. The Wandsworth Heart & Stroke Study. *Clin Sci* 2003; **104**: 591–8.

41. UKPDS group 39. Efficacy of atenolol and captopril in reducing risk of macrovascular and microvascular complications in type 2 diabetes. *Br Med J* 1998; **317**: 713–20.

42. Hansson L, Zanchetti A, Carruthers SG, Dahlof B, Elmfeldt D, Julius S et al. Effects of intensive blood pressure lowering and low-dose aspirin in patients with hypertension: principal results of the hypertension optimal treatment (HOT) randomised trial. *Lancet* 1998; **351**: 1755–62.

43. Executive summary of the Third Report of the National Cholesterol Education Program (NCEP) Expert Panel on Detection, Evaluation and Treatment of High Blood Cholesterol in Adults (Adult Treatment Panel III). *JAMA* 2001; **285**: 2486–97.43.

44. Cappuccio FP, Barbato A, Kerry SM. Hypertension, diabetes and cardiovascular risk in ethnic minorities in the UK. *Br J Diabetes Vasc Dis* 2003; **3**: 286–93.

45. Ness AR, Cappuccio FP, Atkinson RW, Khaw K-T, Cook DG. Plasma vitamin C levels in men and women from different ethnic backgrounds living in England. *Int J Epidemiol* 1999; **28**: 450–5.

46. Kulkarni KR, Markovitz JH, Nanda NC, Segrest JP. Increased prevalence of smaller and denser LDL particles in Asian Indians. *Arterioscler Thromb Vasc Biol* 1999; **19**: 2749–55.

47. Kain K, Catto AJ, Grant PJ. Impaired fibrinolysis and increased fibrinogen levels in South Asian subjects. *Atherosclerosis* 2001; **156**: 457–61.

48. Crook M, Kerai P, Andrews V, Lumb P, Swaminathan R. Serum sialic acid, a reputed cardiovascular risk factor, is elevated in South Asian men compared to European men. *Ann Clin Biochem* 1998; **35**: 242–4.

49. Baker EH, Dong YB, Sagnella GA, Rothwell M, Onipinla AK, Markandu ND et al. Association of hypertension with T594M mutation in b3 subunit of epithelial sodium channels in black people resident in London. *Lancet* 1998; **351**: 1388–92.

50. Dong YB, Zhu HD, Sagnella GA, Carter ND, Cook DG, Cappuccio FP. Association between the C825T polymorphism of the G protein b3 subunit gene and hypertension in blacks. *Hypertension* 1999; **34**: 1193–6.

51. Dong YB, Zhu HD, Baker EH, Sagnella GA, MacGregor GA, Carter ND et al. T594M and G442V polymorphisms of the sodium channel b3 subunit and hypertension in a black population. *J Hum Hypert* 2001; **15**: 425–30.

52. Sagnella GA, Rothwell MJ, Onipinla AK, Wicks PD, Cook DG, Cappuccio FP. A population study of ethnic variations in the angiotensin-converting enzyme I/D polymorphism: relationships with gender, hypertension and impaired glucose metabolism. *J Hypertens* 1999; **17**: 657–64.

53. Hall S, Talmud PJ, Cook DG, Wicks PD, Rothwell MJ, Strazzullo P et al. Frequency and allelic association of common variants in the lipoprotein lipase gene in different ethnic groups. The Wandsworth Heart & Stroke Study. *Gen Epidemiol* 2000; **18**: 203–16.

54. Waterworth DM, Talmud PJ, Humphries SE, Wicks PD, Sagnella GA, Strazzullo P et al. Variable effects of the ApoCIII -482C>T variant on insulin, glucose and triglyceride levels in different ethnic groups. The Wandsworth Heart & Stroke Study. *Diabetologia* 2001; **44**: 245–8.

55. Hayes L, White M, Unwin N, Bhopal R, Fischbacher C, Harland J et al. Patterns of physical activity and relationship with risk markers for cardiovascular disease and diabetes in Indian, Pakistani, Bangladeshi and European adults in a UK population. *J Public Health Med* 2002; **24**: 170–8.

56. Chambers JC, Obeid OA, Refsum H, Ueland P, Hackett D, Hooper J et al. Plasma homocysteine concentrations and risk of coronary heart disease in UK Indian Asian and European men. *Lancet* 2000; **355**: 523–7.

57. Mehrotra S, Ling KL, Bekele Y, Gerbino E, Earle KA. Lipid hydroperoxide and markers of renal disease susceptibility in African-Caribbean and Caucasian patients with type 2 diabetes mellitus. *Diabet Med* 2001; **18**: 109–15.

58. Fischbacher CM, Bhopal R, Rutter MK, Unwin NC, Marshall SM, White M et al. Microalbuminuria is more frequent in South Asian than in European origin populations: a comparative study in Newcastle, UK. *Diabet Med* 2003; **20**: 31–6.

59. Abuaisha B, Kumar S, Malik R, Boulton AJ. Relationship of elevated urinary albumin excretion to components of the metabolic syndrome in non-insulin-dependent diabetes mellitus. *Diabetes Res Clin Pract* 1998; **39**: 93–9.

4
Management strategies for cerebrovascular disease in South Asians

Pankaj Sharma and Simon Korn

Introduction

Stroke is a major cause of disability and the second commonest cause of dementia.[1] UK data show that the standardised mortality ratio (SMR) for cerebrovascular disease amongst the South Asian population of England and Wales is 41% higher in women and 55% higher in men compared to the general population (Table 4.1). Although mortality is decreasing, the rate of decrease in the South Asian community is slower than in the general population.[2] Globally, the third most common cause of death (5.5 million people in 2002 or 10% of all deaths worldwide) is stroke[3] and the mortality and

Table 4.1 Numbers of deaths from cerebrovascular disease (ICD codes 430–438) and standardised mortality ratios (SMR) for total population and selected immigrant groups aged 20–69 years in England and Wales for the periods 1970–2 and 1989–92. (ADAPTED FROM REFERENCE 2)

Country of birth	Period	Men		Women	
		No of deaths	SMR (95% CI)	No of deaths	SMR (95% CI)
Total population	1970–2	31 271	195 (191 to199)	27 428	206 (202– 210)
	1989–92	21 421	100	17 334	100
South Asia	1970–2	244	226 (198–256)	165	246 (210– 286)
	1989–92	594	155 (143–168) *	344	141 (127–157) *
Scotland	1970–2	533	183 (168–199)	425	198 (180–218)
	1989–92	554	125 (115–136)	416	125 (113–137)
Ireland	1970–2	756	234 (154–166)	596	235 (216–254)
	1989–92	758	138 (128–148)	553	123 (113–133)
East Africa	1989–92	56	114 (86–147)	43	122 (88–164)
West Africa	1989–92	67	271 (210–344)	26	181 (118–265)
Caribbean	1970–2	177	394 (338–457)	137	463 (389–547)
	1989–92	360	168 (151–186)	212	157 (136–179)

morbidity caused by stroke is likely to increase as the world's population ages. Hypertension is the most common modifiable risk factor for stroke worldwide. Around 27% of urban dwellers in India are hypertensive compared with just 12% in rural regions.[4] Authoritative opinions for this discrepancy can be found elsewhere but it is clear that such a high prevalence of hypertension will greatly increase the burden of stroke in South Asia. Some comfort may be had in the knowledge that the rates of total cholesterol are lower compared with western populations but since levels of high density lipoprotein (HDL) are also lower, the cholesterol:HDL ratio is often raised. These risk factors are further compounded by higher rates of diabetes in the South Asian population increasing the likelihood of an ischaemic cerebrovascular event. The 10-year risk estimates for stroke in South Asians living in a western society have been shown to be 1.6 (1.5–1.8) compared to white Europeans at 1.4 (1.3–1.6), although those from African descent are the highest at 1.7 (1.5–1.9).[5] Indeed, within western countries there is increasing evidence that there is an excess mortality and morbidity among certain ethnic groups.[6–10] On the Indian subcontinent, where there is observed an increase in risk factors including smoking and the introduction of western lifestyle and dietary habits, the increased burden due to stroke may be particularly severe,[11] and about half the world's cardiovascular burden is predicted to occur in the Asia-Pacific region.[12] However, available epidemiological data from this region is very limited[13] and the increased rates of coronary heart disease (CHD) have been shown to be variable across sections of the South Asian population in the UK.[14–15] The more economically advantaged South Asian group, that is Indians, have rates that are similar to those found among white European people, while the poorest groups, namely Pakistanis and Bangladeshis, have rates that are considerably higher. Socioeconomic position predicts risk in each ethnic group and makes a key contribution to the higher risk found for Pakistani and Bangladeshi individuals.[14]

Mortality amongst ethnic minority populations in the UK

It is well known that the profile of all-cause mortality amongst immigrants to the UK varies with country of origin.[16–17] In particular, the SMR for CHD is higher amongst South Asians than the white European population but lower in people of West African or Caribbean origin.[2] In the case of cerebrovascular events, deaths from all subtypes of stroke tend to occur at a younger age in ethnic minority groups compared to a white European population (Table 4.2). Although all-cause events are greater in South Asians (3.46 per 100 patient years) compared to white Europeans (2.5) and Afro-Caribbean (0.9), the majority of this event rate is made up of coronary events rather than cerebrovascular.[18]

Table 4.2 % death from stroke in subjects under 65 years of age by ethnic group
(ADAPTED FROM: http://www.cdc.gov/cvh/maps/strokeatlas/03-section1.htm)

Ethnic group	(%) Stroke death <65 years age
American Indians & Alaska natives	25
Asians & Pacific Islanders	22
Blacks	27
Hispanics	26
Whites	9

Possible reasons for increased cerebrovascular disease amongst South Asians

The precise mechanisms underlying the excess cerebrovascular mortality in South Asians (Table 4.3)[2] have not been fully explained but may be similar to those underlying the increased risk of cardiac disease (see also Chapter 3). Although the prevalence of classical risk factors is higher in the South Asian population,[15] this is not enough to

Table 4.3 Haemorrhagic and ischaemic stroke type by ethnicity
(ADAPTED FROM: http://www.cdc.gov/cvh/maps/strokeatlas/03-section1.htm)

Ethnic group*	Haemorrhagic (%)	Ischaemic (%)
American Indians & Alaska natives	26	8
Asians & Pacific Islanders	38	8
Blacks	24	10
Hispanics	32	9
Whites	18	11

*Age ≥ 35 years

explain the excess vascular risk. For example, although European Canadians are more likely to have atherosclerosis – a major risk factor – South Asian Canadians are still twice as likely to suffer a stroke or heart attack. Thus, other factors such as insulin resistance[19] may predispose to an increased risk for vascular disease in the South Asian population.

Metabolic syndrome/Insulin resistance syndrome

Several studies suggest that the metabolic syndrome, including insulin resistance,[20] hyperinsulinaemia, higher waist–hip ratio, visceral adiposity,[21] hypertriglyceridaemia, low HDL cholesterol, high lipoprotein(a) levels and a higher prevalence of hypertension may account at least in part for this increased risk.[22–24]

Thrombotic risk factors

It has also been shown that insulin resistance significantly clusters with pro-fibrotic and pro-thrombotic factors in South Asians, for example, increased levels of fibrinogen, von Willebrand factor, tissue plasminogen activator antigen (tPA), plasminogen activator inhibitor (PAI-1), factor XIIa, factor VII antigen and factor XIII B subunit.[25–27] These factors may contribute to the higher prevalence of cerebrovascular disease in South Asians. However, Kain et al (2002)[27] showed that the higher levels of fibrinogen, von Willebrand factor and t-PA in South Asian stroke patients disappeared after adjustment for insulin resistance syndrome. Thus, these changes may only be secondary features of insulin resistant syndrome.[27]

Homocysteine

Homocysteine and the MTHFR C677T mutation are increasingly becoming recognized as a risk factor for stroke.[28–32] This evidence, however, is still based on observational studies or Mendelian randomisation which have their limitations.[33] Notwithstanding this caveat, it has been shown that South Asians[34] and Bangladeshis[35] have higher levels of homocysteine. Dietary factors and vegetarianism may be at least in part responsible for this.[36]

Other potential cerebrovascular risk factors

Other suggested risk factors for an increase in cerebrovascular disease in South Asians include migration, poor diet, lack of exercise, endothelial factors, enhanced inflammation and disadvantaged socioeconomic status.[37] Another possibility is that certain risk factors have an increased potency or interact in a different way in this population group. Certain ethnically specific health-seeking behaviour, health beliefs, communication problems and atypical presentations of illness or interpretation of symptoms may also have an effect.[38–40]

Variations in the management of inpatients with stroke among different ethnic groups

Few studies have investigated differences in clinical management of stroke between different ethnic groups and previous studies have focused on Afro-Caribbean groups and comparison with their white European counterparts.[41–42] A variety of reasons for this paucity of research is proffered not least because controversy still exists surrounding the use of ethnicity and race as variables in medical research.[43–49] Some claim that current terminology overemphasises the homogeneity within groups and the contrast between them and that the complex relationship with socioeconomic factors and racism makes interpretation of results problematic.[2, 50] Others assert that on the basis of the logical premises of observational studies of racial comparisons, aetiological inferences cannot be made.[43] A strict methodological approach to ethnicity such as that used for socio-economic status (which is also a composite measure of income, education, attitudes and beliefs regarding health)[43, 51] is required if the concept of ethnicity is to be clinically useful (i.e. generalisable through time and across cultures).[47] Although the British Medical Journal[52] and the Journal of the American Medical Association[53] have produced some guidelines to address this issue there are still very few journals with a strongly implemented policy on ethnicity/race.[50, 54] In particular, there is a lack of accepted terminology for particular ethnic groups exists and authors rarely explain in detail how subjects are designated into these groups.

Using such strict criteria, our group have attempted to study differences in clinical management of stroke among ethnic groups.[55] The Royal London Hospital, one of the largest hospital Trusts in the UK with over 1,100 beds and serving a catchment population of around 500,000, was studied. This large teaching hospital is based in the inner city and includes a large Bangladeshi community (at higher risk of cerebrovascular disease) within its catchment population. All patients from the Bangladeshi and white European (English, Scottish, Welsh) communities with a diagnosis at discharge of ischaemic stroke were recruited. A total of 265 patients met the inclusion criteria with 186 of British (English, Scottish or Welsh; mean age of stroke onset 66 years) and the remainder of Bangladeshi ancestry (mean age 62 years). Simple measurement of cholesterol levels was much more likely to have been performed in Caucasians (76%) compared to Bangladeshis (25%). Although neuroimaging (CT/MRI) and echocardiography were more likely to be performed in the Bangladeshi cohort compared to white Europeans, there were no differences in undertaking carotid imaging (MRA and/or Doppler studies). There were no significant differences in either referral patterns or intervention for carotid endarterectomy. Only 34% of all patients were discharged on lipid-lowering drugs (36% Caucasians; 29% Bangladeshis). White Europeans were more likely to be started on warfarin (8%) compared to Bangladeshis (1.3%) which may be explained by the greater incidence of atrial fibrillation (AF) in the former group. Our study showed that there were differences in the clinical management of stroke in the Bangladeshi compared with the white European population, although the management of stroke in both groups was poor.

Only one other study[56] has been conducted in the UK which has examined trends involving stroke management in groups from the Indian subcontinent. The investigators found that South Asian stroke patients were less likely to be admitted acutely to hospital when compared with their white European counterparts. This study, similar to many involving ethnicity, made no attempt to further sub-define the South Asian population. This paucity of definition is important because of emerging data that subgroups within the South Asian population, e.g. Bangladeshis, have differing risk profile in terms of vascular disease compared to other Asians.[57]

The reasons for the failure of exemplary stroke management in Bangladeshis are probably diverse and are likely to include lack of translation facilities (an important factor well recognised by previous studies[58]), late presentation of disease, differences in case mix and cultural misunderstanding rather than wilful differential treatment.

Conclusion

There is growing evidence that certain ethnic groups are at higher risk of cerebrovascular disease than others. Although most of the attention in South Asians has been on CHD, it is now increasingly clear that South Asians are also at a greater risk of cerebrovascular disease and that amongst South Asians, Bangladeshis are most at risk. Primary and secondary prevention strategies for the general population need to be improved and the need amongst those at higher risk is more pressing. Some argue that guidelines need to be adapted to the target population and that the threshold for initiating treatment when absolute risk may be underestimated should be lowered.[59] Another issue is the need for 'cultural competence' when addressing inequities in health and provision of health services.[60] Further research on ethnicity and stroke may reveal more about the pathophysiology of cerebrovascular disease and lead to more effective treatment and targeted interventions. What is clear is that the research on stroke in South Asians is almost non-existent and this is a situation that is untenable.

Update from the Department of Health

The National Audit Office (NAO), the organisation which scrutinises public spending on behalf of Parliament, has produced a report looking at whether the NHS is providing effective and high quality stroke care services in England and whether the Department of Health is managing and supporting the programme of stroke care well. The report shows that notable progress has been made from a low starting point and recommends further improvements in stroke prevention and treating and managing stroke patients, in line with recent evidence. Although the report did not specifically look at stroke services for the South Asian communities its analysis and recommendations will be relevant to the management of all stroke patients.

In response to the NAO report the Department of Health has announced that work will begin on a new stroke strategy which will deliver the newest treatments and improve the care that stroke patients receive. Early action will include spreading examples of best practice and will build a future generation of clinical champions through a programme to expand stroke physician training numbers. There is a new policy team specifically for stroke, recently established at the Department of Health, which will drive this work forward.[61]

The Department is keen to improve public awareness of stroke amongst all groups. Low public awareness of stroke – symptoms and prevention – is one of the areas highlighted in the NAO report. To help raise awareness and encourage people to treat stroke as a medical emergency the Department has drafted a set of key messages (see Annex A) for organisations to use and promote with a consistent form of words.

References

1. The World Health Organisation. The Atlas of Heart Disease and Stroke. http://www.who.in/cardiovascular_diseases/en/cvd_atlas_16_death_from_stroke.pdf

2. Wild S, McKeigue P. Cross sectional analysis of mortality by country of birth in England and Wales, 1970–92. *Br Med J* 1997; **314**: 705.

3. Asia Pacific Consensus Forum on Stroke Management. *Stroke* 1998; **29**(8): 1730–6.

4. Nath I, Reddy KS, Dinshaw KA, Bhisey AN, Krishnaswami K et al. Country Profile: India. *Lancet* 1998; **351**; 1265–75.

5. Cappuccio FP, Oakeshott P, Strazzullo P, Kerry SM. Application of Framingham risk estimates to ethnic minorities in United Kingdom and implications for primary prevention of heart disease in general practice: cross sectional population based study. *Br Med J* 2002; **325**: 1271.

6. Stroke epidemiological data of nine Asian countries. Asian Acute Stroke Advisory Panel (AASAP). *Med Assoc Thai* 2000; **83**(1): 1–7.

7. Chaturvedi N, Fuller JH. Ethnic differences in mortality from cardiovascular disease in the UK: do they persist in people with diabetes? *J Epidemiol Community Health* 1996; **50**(2): 137–9.

8. White H, Boden-Albala B, Wang C, Elkind MS, Rundek T, Wright CB, Sacco RL. Ischemic stroke subtype incidence among whites, blacks, and Hispanics: the Northern Manhattan Study. *Circulation* 2005; **111**(10): 1327–31.

9. Ayala C, Greenlund KJ, Croft JB, Keenan NL, Donehoo RS, Giles WH, Kittner SJ, Marks JS. Racial/ethnic disparities in mortality by stroke subtype in the United States, 1995–1998. *Am J Epidemiol* 2001; **154**(11):1057–63.

10. Nath I, Reddy KS, Dinshaw KA, Bhisey AN, Krishnaswami K, Bhan MK, Ganguly NK, Kaur S, Panda SK, Jameel S, Srinivasan K, Thankappan KR, Valiathan MS. Country profile: India. *Lancet* 1998; **351**(9111): 1265–75.

11. Casper ML, Barnett E, Williams GI Jr., Halverson JA, Braham VE, Greenlund KJ. *Atlas of Stroke Mortality: Racial, Ethnic, and Geographic Disparities in the United States.* Atlanta, GA: Department of Health and Human Services, Centers for Disease Control and Prevention, 2003. http://www.cdc.gov/cvh/maps/strokeatlas/03-section1.htm

12. 2001 Oregon State of the Heart and Stroke Report. Race and Ethnicity Prevalence and Risk Factors. http://oregon.gov/DHS/ph/hdsp/2001/race.shtml

13. Cooper RS, Kaufman JS. Race and hypertension: science and nescience. *Hypertension* 1998; **32**(5): 813–6.

14. Nazroo JY. South Asian people and heart disease: an assessment of the importance of socioeconomic position. *Ethnic Dis* 2001; **11**(3): 401–11.

15. Razaaq AA, Khan BA, Baig SM. Ischaemic stroke in young adults of South Asia. *J Pak Med Assoc* 2002; **52**(9): 417–22.

16. Marmot MG, Adelstein AM, Bulusu L. *Immigrant mortality in England and Wales 1970–78: causes of death by country of birth.* London: HMSO 1984. (OPCS studies on medical and population subjects No 47.)

17. Balarajan R, Bulusu L. Mortality among immigrants in England and Wales, 1979–83. In: Briton M (ed). *Mortality and Geography. A review in the mid 1980s. England and Wales.* London: HMSO 1990: 103–21. (OPCS series DS No 9.)

18. Khattar RS, Swales JD, Senior R, and Lahiri A. Racial variation in cardiovascular morbidity and mortality in essential hypertension. *Heart* 2000; **83**: 267–271.

19. Kain K, Catto AJ, Young J, Bamford J, Bavington J, Grant PJ. Insulin Resistance and Elevated Levels of Tissue Plasminogen Activator in First-Degree Relatives of South Asian Patients with Ischemic Cerebrovascular Disease. *Stroke* 2001; **32**: 1069–1073.

20. Kernan WN, Inzucchi SE, Viscoli CM, Brass LM, Bravata DM, Horwitz RI. Insulin resistance and risk for stroke. *Neurology* 2002; **59**: 809–815.

21. Raji A, Seely EW, Arky RA, Simonson DC. Body fat distribution and insulin resistance in healthy Asian Indians and Caucasians. *J Clin Endocrinol Metab* 2001; **86**(11): 5366–71.

22. Anand SS, Yusuf S, Vuksan V, Devanesen S, Teo KK, Montague PA, Kelemen L, Yi C, Lonn E, Gerstein H, Hegele RA. Differences in risk factors, atherosclerosis and cardiovascular disease between ethnic groups in Canada: the study of health assessment and risk in ethnic groups (SHARE). *Indian Heart J* 2000; **52**(7 Suppl): S35–43.

23. Dhawan J, Bray CL, Warburton R, Ghambhir D, Morris J. Insulin resistance, high prevalence of diabetes, and cardiovascular risk in immigrant Asians: genetic or environmental effect? *Br Heart J* 1994; **72**: 413–421.

24. McKeigue PM, Ferrie JE, Pierpoint T, Marmot MG. Association of early-onset coronary heart disease in South Asian men with glucose intolerance and hyperinsulinemia. *Circulation* 1993; **87**: 152–161.

25. Kain K, Catto AJ, Grant PJ. Associations between insulin resistance and thrombotic risk factors in high-risk South Asian subjects. *Diabet Med* 2003; **20**(8): 651–5.

26. Kain K, Catto AJ, Grant PJ. Clustering of thrombotic factors with insulin resistance in South Asian patients with ischaemic stroke. *Thromb Haemost* 2002; **88**(6): 950–3.

27. Kain K, Catto AJ, Young J, Bamford J, Bavington J, Grant PJ. Increased fibrinogen, von Willebrand factor and tissue plasminogen activator levels in insulin resistant South Asian patients with ischaemic stroke. *Atherosclerosis* 2002; **163**(2): 371–6.

28. Casas JP, Bautista LE, Smeeth L, Sharma P, Hingorani AD. Homocysteine and stroke: evidence on a causal link from mendelian randomisation. *Lancet* 2005; **15**: 365:224–32.

29. Cronin S, Furie KL, Kelly PJ. Dose-Related Association of MTHFR 677T Allele With Risk of Ischemic Stroke. Evidence From a Cumulative Meta-Analysis. *Stroke* 2005; **36**: 1581–1587.

30. Kelly PJ, Rosand J, Kistler JP et al. Homocysteine, MTHFR 677CT polymorphism, and risk of ischemic stroke: results of a meta-analysis. *Neurology* 2002; **59**: 529–536.

31. Boysen G, Brander T, Christensen H, Gideon R and Truelsen T. Homocysteine and Risk of Recurrent Stroke. *Stroke* 2003; **34**(5): 1258–1261.

32. Boushey CJ, Beresford SA, Omenn GS et al. A quantitative assessment of plasma homocysteine as a risk factor for vascular disease: probable benefits of increasing folic acid intake. *JAMA* 1995; **274**: 1049–1057.

33. Minelli C, Thompson JR, Tobin MD, and Abrams KR. An Integrated Approach to the Meta-Analysis of Genetic Association Studies using Mendelian Randomization. *Am J Epidemiol* 2004; **160**: 445–452.

34. Carmel R, Mallidi PV, Vinarskiy S, Brar S, Frouhar Z. Hyperhomocysteinemia and cobalamin deficiency in young Asian Indians in the United States. *Am J Hematol* 2002; **70**(2): 107–14.

35. Gamble MV, Ahsan H, Liu X, Factor-Litvak P, Ilievski V, Slavkovich V, Parvez F, Graziano JH. Folate and cobalamin deficiencies and hyperhomocysteinemia in Bangladesh. *Am J Clin Nutr* 2005; **81**(6): 1372–7.

36. Cappuccio FP, Bell R, Perry IJ, Gilg J, Ueland PM, Refsum H, Sagnella GA, Jeffery S, Cook DG. Homocysteine levels in men and women of different ethnic and cultural background living in England. *Atherosclerosis* 2002; **164**(1): 95–102.

37. Velmurugan C, Kuppuswamy, Gupta S. Excess coronary heart disease in South Asians in the United Kingdom. *Br Med J* 2005; **330**: 1223–1224.

38. Lawton J, Ahmad N, Hallowell N, Hanna L, Douglas M. Perceptions and experiences of taking oral hypoglycaemic agents among people of Pakistani and Indian origin: qualitative study. *Br Med J* 2005; **330**: 1247.

39. Shaikh BT, Hatcher J. Health seeking behaviour and health service utilization in Pakistan: challenging the policy makers. *J Public Health* 2005; **27**: 49–54.

40. Barakat K, Wells Z, Ramdhany S, Mills PG, Timmis AD. Bangladeshi patients present with non-classic features of acute myocardial infarction and are treated less aggressively in east London, UK. *Heart* 2003; **89**: 276–9.

41. Stewart JA, Dundas R, Howard RS, Rudd AG, Wolfe CD: Ethnic differences in incidence of stroke: prospective study with stroke register. *Br Med J* 1999; **318**: 967–971

42. Wolfe CD, Rudd AG, Howard R, Coshall C, Stewart J, Lawrence E, Hajat C, Hillen T. Incidence and case fatality rates of stroke subtypes in a multiethnic population: the South London Stroke Register. *J Neurol Neurosurg Psychiatry* 2002; **72**: 211–216

43. Chaturvedi N. Ethnicity as an epidemiological determinant – crudely racist or crucially important? *Int J Epidemiol* 2001; **30**(5): 925–7.

44. Osbourne NG, Feit MD. The use of race in medical research. *J Am Med Assoc* 1992; **267**: 275–79.

45. Sheldon T, Parker H. Race and ethnicity in health research. *J Public Health Med* 1992; **14(2)**: 104–10.

46. Senior PA, Bhopal R. Ethnicity as a variable in epidemiological research. *Br Med J* 1994; **309**: 327–30.

47. Witzig R. The Medicalization of Race: Scientific Legitimization of a Flawed Social Construct. *Ann Intern Med* 1996; **125**(8): 675 – 679.

48. Bhopal R. Is research into ethnicity and health racist, unsound, or important science? *Br Med J* 1997; **314**: 1751–1751.

49. Gamble VN. Under the shadow of Tuskegee: African Americans and health care. *Am J Public Health* 1997; **87**: 1773–78.

50. Bhopal R. Glossary of terms relating to ethnicity and race: for reflection and debate. *J Epidemiol Community Health* 2004; **58**(6): 441 – 445.

51. Senior PA, Bhopal R. Ethnicity as a variable in epidemiological research. *Br Med J* 1994; **309**: 327–330.

52. Anonymous. Ethnicity, race and culture: guidelines for research, audit and publication. *Br Med J* 1996; **312**: 1094.

53. Kaplan JB, Bennett T. Use of Race and Ethnicity in Biomedical Publication. *JAMA* 2003; **289**: 2709–2716.

54. Bhopal R, Rankin J, Bennett T. Editorial Role in Promoting Valid Use of Concepts and Terminology in Race and Ethnicity Research http://www.councilscienceeditors.org/members/securedDocuments/v23n3p075-080.pdf

55. Bourke J, Sylvester R, Sharma P. Ethnic variations in the management of patients with acute stroke. Postgrad. *Med J* (*in press*)

56. Hsu RT, Ardron ME, Brooks W, Cherry D, Taub NA, Botha JL. The 1996 Leicestershire Community Stroke & Ethnicity Study: differences and similarities between South Asian and white strokes. *Int J Epidemiol* 1999; **28**: 853–858.

57. Bhopal R, Unwin N, White M, Yallop J, Walker L, Alberti KG, Harland J, Patel S, Ahmad N, Turner C, Watson B, Kaur D, Kulkarni A, Laker M, Tavridou A. Heterogeneity of coronary heart disease risk factors in Indian, Pakistani, Bangladeshi, and European origin populations: cross sectional study. *Br Med J* 1999; **319**: 215–20.

58. Gerrish K. The nature and effect of communication difficulties arising from interactions between district nurses and South Asian patients and their carers. *J Adv Nurs* 2001; **33**: 566–574.

59. Cappuccio FP, Oakeshott P, Strazzullo P, Kerry SM. Application of Framingham risk estimates to ethnic minorities in United Kingdom and implications for primary prevention of heart disease in general practice: cross sectional population based study. *Br Med J* 2002; **325**: 1271.

60. Betancourt JR, Green AR, Carrillo JE, Aneneh-Firempong O. Defining cultural competence: a practical framework for addressing racial/ethnic disparities in health and health care. *Public Health Rep* 2003; **118**: 293–302.

61. For more information contact Anna Norris on 0207 972 3042.

Annex A   Stroke Key Messages

What you need to know about … strokes

What is a stroke?

- A stroke is a brain attack. It happens when the blood supply to the brain is disrupted.
- There are two types of stroke.
- Most strokes occur when a blood clot blocks the flow of blood to the brain. Some strokes are caused by bleeding in or around the brain from a burst blood vessel.
- In both cases the brain is starved of oxygen, damaging or killing cells.
- Sufferers are often left with difficulty talking, walking and performing other basic tasks.

How can I improve my lifestyle to reduce my risk of having a stroke?

You can reduce the risk of having a stroke (as well as heart disease, cancer and diabetes) by making the following lifestyle changes:

- Stop smoking.
- Reduce alcohol consumption.
- Eat a healthy diet. This means reducing your salt intake, eating lots of fruit, vegetables, wholegrain foods and fish, and less fat, red and processed meat.
- Take regular exercise and try to keep a healthy weight.
- Maintain the right blood pressure and low cholesterol levels.

What are the symptoms of a stroke?

Not everyone will have the same symptoms and the symptoms may vary. The most common symptoms to look out for are:

- A sudden weakness or numbness of the face, arm or leg on one side of the body.
- Sudden loss or blurring of vision, in one or both eyes.
- Sudden difficulty speaking or understanding spoken language.

- Sudden confusion.
- Sudden or severe headache with no apparent cause.
- Dizziness, unsteadiness or a sudden fall, especially with any of the other symptoms.

What are the clear signs that someone has had a stroke?

- Facial weakness. Can the person smile? Has their mouth or eye drooped?
- Arm weakness. Can the person raise both arms?
- Speech problems. Can the person speak clearly and understand what you say?

What should I do if I think someone has had a stroke?

- A stroke is a medical emergency. If you suspect a stroke call 999 immediately.
- By calling 999, you can help someone reach hospital quickly and receive the early treatment they need.
- Prompt action can prevent further damage to the brain and help someone make a full recovery.
- Delay can result in death or major long-term disabilities like paralysis, severe memory loss and communication problems.

What is a Transient Ischaemic Attack or TIA?

- A TIA (sometimes called mini stroke) is similar to a full stroke but the symptoms may only last a few minutes and will have completely gone within 24 hours.
- Don't ignore this because it could lead to a major stroke.
- See your GP as soon as possible and ask to be referred to a specialist stroke service. This should happen within seven days.

Where can I get further information?

NHS Direct On-line: www.nhsdirect.nhs.uk

The Stroke Association: www.stroke.org.uk
Helpline: 0845 303 3100

Men's Health Forum: www.malehealth.co.uk

5
The challenge of cardiac rehabilitation in South Asians

Nam Sahni and Rosalind Leslie

Introduction

Coronary Heart Disease (CHD) remains the most common cause of premature death in the UK. In South Asians, as discussed in previous chapters, the rates are approximately 50% higher. Whilst mortality rates from CHD in the UK have declined over the last few decades in the general population, mortality rates in South Asian populations have not shown a similar trend,[1] particularly in the younger age groups.[2] This perhaps demonstrates that CHD prevention strategies which are successful for the general population fail to have a similar impact in South Asian populations, underlining the need for more research and education in this area.

Cardiac rehabilitation is often recommended following acute myocardial infarction, coronary artery bypass graft or angioplasty as it is a clinically useful method of modifying CHD risk factors. In 1993, the World Health Organisation[3] defined the rehabilitation of cardiac patients as 'the sum of activities required to influence favourably the underlining cause of the disease, as well as the best possible physical, mental and social conditions, so that they may preserve or resume, when lost, as normal a place as possible in the community. Rehabilitation cannot be regarded as an isolated form of therapy, but must be integrated with the whole treatment of which it forms only one facet.'

The benefits of cardiac rehabilitation programmes are well documented, with evidence demonstrating measurable benefits on morbidity and mortality,[4] but there are relatively little data specific to cardiac rehabilitation provision and benefits for women, the elderly and minority ethnic groups. Uptake of cardiac rehabilitation services in the UK generally ranges from 30% to 59%.[5] However, data indicate that women and elderly and minority ethnic patient groups enrol in cardiac rehabilitation programmes at a significantly lower rate than white middle-aged men,[6] but those patients who do attend exercise training programmes derive benefit.[7] We describe in this review our experience in developing cardiovascular rehabilitation services for South Asian patients in Wolverhampton (UK), a region where a significant proportion of the population served is from this ethnic group.

What are the challenges?

There are many barriers to equitable delivery of and benefit from cardiac rehabilitation programmes in South Asians. Some of the more common and significant challenges in the quest to modify risk factors in South Asian patients include:

- Barriers to communication
- Reduced healthcare professional awareness of dietary habits
- Low levels of physical activity
- Cultural issues
- High levels of comorbidity
- Nihilistic attitudes

Initiatives developed in Wolverhampton to address such issues include:

- Appointment of a CHD Asian Link Nurse
- Production of audio cassettes containing healthy lifestyle advice and local cardiac rehabilitation information in Punjabi
- Women-only exercise sessions

A high percentage of South Asian patients suffer from more than one disease process and have several cardiovascular risk factors.[8] For example, diabetes, a potent risk factor for CHD in South Asians, is three to five times more common in people of South Asian origin living in the UK and often coexists with obesity and physical inactivity. This complicates the task of educating this group about their medical conditions and derivation of a tailored management plan.

The largest challenge, perhaps, is comprehension of education. Practitioners are often unsure about comprehension of information given to the patient and their carers. However, the availability of multilingual literature is now increasing, e.g. from the British Heart Foundation, Diabetes UK and the South Asian Health Foundation. In the absence of illiteracy (yet another challenge to rehabilitation services), such provision of literature is an important and necessary step in the delivery of culturally appropriate services.

Fatalistic and episodic approaches to health and illness have been highlighted by health professionals as being characteristics of South Asian patients, and influence patient behaviour when ill and suffering from chronic conditions.[9] South Asians are great believers in destiny and fate, often quoting 'this is God's will' or 'what is written in my destiny no-one can change'. Such an approach to health often results in patients being less proactive in the recovery process. Due to this fatalistic approach to life, Asians quickly shift into a 'disabled' role. To overcome such behaviour and beliefs is a major challenge. Any attempt to alter cognition would have to be approached sensitively and with informed consideration of both religious and cultural issues. There is a challenge, not only to induce patients to grasp a basic understanding of their disease process, but then subsequently to encourage adoption of a healthier lifestyle, a concept which may be met with strong resistance or even refusal.

The most important predictors of outcome and compliance are patients' beliefs about the cause and course of their disease and the number of misconceptions held.[10] Health care professionals and patients may not share the same beliefs about the cause and course of illness. Therefore, professionals must take on the responsibility for identifying the belief systems of patients. The motives of the health care professional are based on a positive holistic health model, whereas cultural perception is often very pessimistic.

Modifiable risk factors

The prevalence of modifiable risk factors such as smoking, dyslipidaemia and hypertension is generally lower in South Asians than in white Europeans, as described by other authors in this text. However, comparisons between migrant South Asians and non-migrant relatives living in India indicate that the former have significantly higher cholesterol, blood pressure, smoking rates and body mass index, suggesting that the threshold for 'normality' in the general population may indeed be too high for South Asians.[11] Only recently has the scientific community recognised this and facilitated the development of lower 'normal' ranges for biometric variables such as body mass index[12] and dyslipidaemia.[13] This work will inevitably continue over the coming years. For South Asian patients, particularly, attention should be paid to high triglyceride concentrations, low high-density lipoprotein cholesterol (HDL) levels, increased visceral fat (central obesity), hyperinsulinaemia, diabetes and physical inactivity.[14] Insulin resistance and its metabolic consequences are more prevalent in UK South Asians than white Europeans, as discussed by Barnett et al in the next chapter. Effective secondary prevention requires identification of all modifiable risk factors, as they combine to provide a potent risk factor profile in South Asians, with high cardiovascular event rates.

Diet

Diets for the various South Asian groups may be perceived as healthier than the average UK diet. However, fat intake is higher in South Asians born in the UK compared to those who are non-UK born.[15, 16] There are two potential disadvantages for the heart in the classical South Asian diet. Firstly, clarified butter or ghee is a highly valued food used in cooking even by most vegetarians. The 'best' ghee is almost 100% saturated fat, but 'lesser quality' ghee may still have more than 50% saturated fat. Secondly, other than Bangladeshis, South Asians tend to have low levels of fish consumption, particularly oily fish which contain beneficial omega-3 polyunsaturated fatty acids.

Dietary advice is extremely important, especially if there is a high consumption of saturated fat. A positive approach is needed to promote the benefits and advantages of a healthy and traditional South Asian diet. Personal experience has highlighted that talking to South Asian communities and teaching them about alternative cooking methods as well as reinforcing general healthy eating advice has a positive and successful outcome. A practical means of promoting a healthier lifestyle is to encourage the reduction of the use of fat and oil used in cooking, and reducing the consumption of Indian snacks and sweetmeats, which are notoriously high in sugar and fat content.

The family plays an important role when it comes to dietary advice, since most food for South Asian family mealtimes is prepared from basic and fresh ingredients at home. Several projects around the country now focus on the delivery of culturally sensitive dietary advice for South Asians, e.g. the Coventry 5-a-day scheme, Birmingham Food Net, Coriander Club of Spitalfields, etc.[17] Such projects provide an invaluable insight into successful strategies at driving dietary change in South Asians and provide useful models for delivering culturally sensitive rehabilitation and preventative dietary advice.

Exercise

Change of any kind is not always easily accepted. Trying to educate and encourage patients of the benefits of increased physical activity poses a particular challenge. It is well established that compared with the general population South Asian males and females are less likely to take part in physical activity.[18] Dhawan and Bray[19] compared physical activity levels of two groups of CHD patients, UK South Asians and South Asians in India. UK South Asians were more sedentary, with their counterparts in India being significantly more physically active. In both groups, physical activity was associated with a reduction of serum insulin, body mass index and triglyceride levels, and a favourable effect on blood pressure. Indeed, it is likely that low levels of physical activity aggravate hyperinsulinaemia and other disturbances associated with the metabolic syndrome in British Asians. Activities such as walking and supervised cardiac rehabilitation exercise programmes, which provide the recommended levels of physical activity, should be promoted. An example of this is the successful 'Walking for Health' led–walks in Wolverhampton that were launched by the Health Action Zone.[17] Local authorities should be sensitive to the needs of South Asians when encouraging them to use local sports facilities, and recognise that exercise can be linked to activities that are culturally more acceptable. For example, many South Asian females do not use sports facilities as the majority are mixed-sex facilities. This barrier may be easily overcome by arranging separate exercise sessions for females. 'Low-key' activities such as walking can be successfully encouraged in any setting. Another example of a simple educational measure to increase access to facilities is to spread awareness among both staff and users of swimming pools that traditional swimming costumes are not essential.

How do we facilitate change?

Project Dil, based in Leicester,[20] is a good example of culturally sensitive strategies aimed at reducing CHD among South Asians. Results of focus group analysis and interviews showed that South Asians have a range of attitudes to and different levels of knowledge of lifestyle risk factors for CHD. Identified barriers to improving lifestyle with respect to diet and exercise included lack of information (for example, how to cook traditional Asian food more healthily) and cultural barriers such as lack of access to leisure facilities for women. Mental stress directly relevant to ethnic minority status was also perceived as an important cause of CHD, for example loss of the extended family, and children leaving home. Language was identified as a key barrier to accessing health education too.

Cardiac rehabilitation professionals should address each of these barriers, and interventions should be tailored to the individual. The most recent evidence supports a menu-based approach, using appropriate health education tools. Menu-based programmes are flexible and take into account disease complexity. Cardiac rehabilitation staff should be skilled in methods of advising change to the varied South Asian cultural lifestyles, and providing patients with the information and support that they need to make decisions. Patients should be encouraged to take ownership of their own risk factor management, focusing on correction of classical risk factors such as cigarette smoking, dyslipidaemia and hypertension combined with intensive glycaemic control and control of obesity.

The most commonly adopted model in cardiac rehabilitation for facilitating and maintaining change is the transtheoretical model of Prochaska and DiClemente.[21] This particular tool is used to determine where in the cycle of change an individual is placed in relation to a specific behaviour. The role of the cardiac rehabilitation professional is to support behavioural change, taking into account perceived barriers to initiating this change. Appropriate interventions should be used specific to each stage of change.

Psychological models used in rehabilitation

There are several psychological models that have been shown to be effective for initiating behavioural change. Cognitive behavioural therapy addresses the individual's core beliefs and behaviour, helping them to identify dysfunctional thoughts and beliefs, and providing a structured approach to managing change in behaviour. Motivational interviewing helps to empower individuals to reach a decision to change. This technique is particularly useful for individuals who are ambivalent or reluctant to change.

It is helpful to involve key family members in the rehabilitation process.[22] Living in an extended family has advantages and disadvantages. There is an inbuilt social support system and decisions about lifestyle, including diet and exercise, are shared rather than the decision having to be taken individually. Family members should be involved in the information-sharing process in order to prevent misunderstanding about what the patient is capable of and expected to do, and to avoid adopting excessive illness behaviour.

Conclusion

Health care professionals involved in cardiac rehabilitation have a responsibility to provide appropriate and effective services to all patients, regardless of age, gender or ethnicity. Assessment and plans of care should include interventions that are individualised and not simply disease-specific. Cardiac rehabilitation teams and services should work towards meeting the needs of South Asian patients with CHD in ways that are culturally, religiously and linguistically appropriate. Also, the needs of these populations are dynamic. Health behaviours in second and third generation migrants seem to be changing, with smoking rates and dietary intakes becoming acultured and converging towards those of the general population. This will pose a serious challenge in the future as it may result in very different disease risks. The new challenge for cardiac rehabilitation is to ensure that the service responds to these changes as they arise.

References

1. Wilkinson P, Sayer J, Laji K, Grundy C, Marchant B, Kopleman P, Timmis AD. Comparison of case fatality in South Asian and white patients after acute myocardial infarction: observational study. *Br Med J* 1996; **312**: 1330–1333.

2. Chaturvedi N. Ethnic differences in Cardiovascular Disease. *Heart* 2003; **89**: 681–686.

3. World Health Organisation (1993). *Needs and action priorities in Cardiac Rehabilitation and secondary prevention in patients with Coronary Heart Disease.* WHO Technical Report Service 831, WHO Regional Office for Europe, Geneva.

4. O'Connor GT, Buring GE, Yusuf S et al. An overview of randomised trials of rehabilitation with exercise after myocardial infarction. *Circulation* 1989; **80**: 234–44.

5. Thompson P. A review of behavioural change theories in patient compliance to exercise-based rehabilitation following acute myocardial infarction. *Coronary Heart Care* 1999; **3**: 18–24.

6. Thompson DR, Bowman GS, Kitson AL, de Bono DP, Hopkins A. Cardiac rehabilitation services in England and Wales: a national survey. *Int J Cardiol* 1997; **59** (3): 299–304.

7. Tod AM, Wadsworth E, Asif S, Gerrish K. Cardiac rehabilitation: the needs of South Asian cardiac patients. *Br J Nurs* 2001; **10** (16): 1028–33.

8. Simmons D, Williams DRR and Powell MJ. The Coventry Diabetes study: prevalence of diabetes and impaired glucose tolerance in Europids and Asians. *Quarterly Journal of Medicine* 1991; **81**: 1021–1030.

9. Jayaratnam R. Black and ethnic minorities – cultural awareness. London: Newham Health Authority 1990.

10. Lewin B, Robertson IH, Cay EL et al. Effects of self-help myocardial infarction rehabilitation on psychological adjustment and use of health services. *Lancet* 1992; **339**: 1036–1040.

11. Kooner JS. Coronary heart disease in UK Indian Asians: the potential for reducing mortality. *Heart* 1997; **78**: 530–532.

12. International Diabetes Institute (World Health Organization). Co-sponsored by the Regional Office for the Western Pacific, WHO, International Association for the Study of Obesity and the International Obesity Task Force. The Asia-Pacific Perspective: redefining obesity and its treatment. Sydney: Health Communications Australia 2000.

13. South Asian Health Foundation Consensus statement for statin use in South Asians 2004. From www.sahf.org.uk

14. Lip GY, Cader MZ, Lee F, Munir SM, Beevers DG. Ethnic differences in pre-admission levels of physical activity in patients admitted with myocardial infarction. *Int J of Cardiol* 1996; **56**: 169–175.

15. Kooner J and Chambers JC. Conceptualising the causes of coronary heart disease in South Asians. In: Patel KCR and Bhopal RS (eds). *The epidemic of coronary heart disease in South Asian populations: Causes and consequences*. SAHF Publishers 2004.

16. Sanders TAB. Nutrition and coronary heart disease in South Asians. In: Patel KCR and Bhopal RS (eds). *The epidemic of coronary heart disease in South Asian populations: Causes and consequences*. SAHF Publishers 2004.

17. Fox C. Heart disease and South Asians: Delivering the National Service Framework for Coronary Heart Disease. NHS 2004.

18. White M. Physical activity among South Asians in Britain. In: Patel KCR and Bhopal RS (eds). *The epidemic of coronary heart disease in South Asian populations: Causes and consequences*. SAHF Publishers 2004.

19. Dhawan J and Bray CL. Asian Indians, coronary artery disease and physical exercise. *Heart* 1997; **78**: 550–554.

20. Farooqi A and Bhavsar M. Project Dil: A co-ordinated Primary Care and community health promotion programme for reducing risk factors for Coronary Heart Disease, amongst the South Asian Community in Leicester. Project Report. November 2000.

21. Prochaska JO and DiClemente CC. Stages and process of self-change of smoking: Toward an integrative model of change. *Journal of Consulting and Clinical Psychology* 1984; **51**: 390–395.

22. Kuppuswamy V, Jhuree K, Gupta S. Coronary artery disease in South Asian prevention (CADISAP) study: a culturally sensitive cardiac rehabilitation (CR): can it improve uptake and adherence of CR among South Asians? *Heart* 2004; 90 (suppl II: abstract 177; A51).

6
Diabetes and cardiovascular disease in UK South Asians: challenges and solutions

Anthony H Barnett, Anthony Dixon and Srikanth Bellary

Introduction

There is now strong evidence that the prevalence of both type 2 diabetes[1–4] (Figure 6.1) and cardiovascular disease (CVD)[5–8] is significantly increased in the South Asian population living in the UK and indeed in many other countries. Statistics suggest that the risk of type 2 diabetes is increased between 4 and 6 fold in this population compared with the corresponding indigenous white European population.[1–4] Standardised mortality rate (SMR) data inform that this is around 150 (i.e. 50% increased SMR) respectively, for both sexes, compared with the general population of England and Wales. Most of the excess mortality is explained on the basis of increased risk of ischaemic heart disease and type 2 diabetes. Women are proportionally more affected than men so that the sex difference in coronary mortality is less in the South Asian compared with the white European population in the UK.[3]

Not only are mortality rates higher in the South Asian population, principally from ischaemic heart disease, but much of the excess risk occurs relatively early.[3] In one study of patients who survived a first myocardial infarction, the average age in South Asians at the time of infarction was around 50 years compared with around 56 years in people of white European origin.[9] In addition, the excess risk appears to be seen in all South Asian populations studied in the UK i.e. those with ancestral origins in Bangladesh, Pakistan, Sri Lanka and India.[8] The increased cardiovascular risk also seems to apply to second generation immigrants in the UK and the impact of an ageing Asian population is likely to make the problem even worse in coming decades.[10]

Studies of rates of coronary heart disease (CHD) in migrant countries compared with South Asians living on the Indian subcontinent are, to an extent, confounded by limited data and geographical distribution but do suggest that urbanisation is critical to the

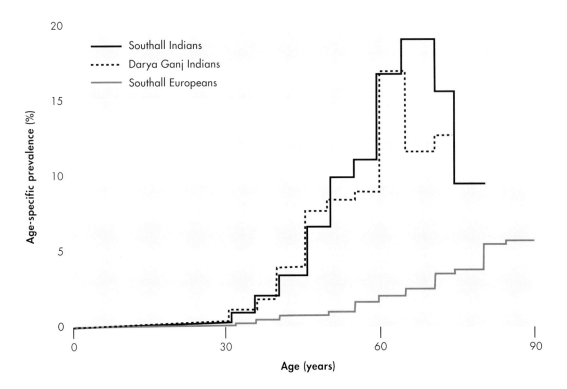

Figure 6.1 Prevalence of diabetes in South Asians living in the UK (Southall Study) and urban India (Darya Ganj Study) compared with the white European population (Southall Study).
ADAPTED AND REPRINTED WITH PERMISSION FROM BLACKWELL SCIENCE. SOURCE: CRUICKSHANK K, PICKUP J, WILLIAMS G, EDS. TEXTBOOK OF DIABETES, SECOND EDITION, VOLUME 1, OXFORD, UK: BLACKWELL SCIENCE LTD; 1997:3.21,FIG 3.10. DATA FROM MATHER HM, KEEN H. *BRIT MED J* 1985; 291:1081–4 AND VERMA NP, MEHTA SP, MADHU S ET AL. BRIT MED J 1986;293:423–4

increased risk of CVD in this population, rather than simply migration *per se.*[3,8] Indeed, people of South Asian origin living in cities in the subcontinent have much higher rates of CHD compared with rural-living populations.[3,8]

In this review we briefly examine the possible reasons for increases in both type 2 diabetes and CVD in the UK South Asian population. We also describe a community-based programme in Birmingham and Coventry which tries to address some of these issues.

Insulin resistance, type 2 diabetes and cardiovascular risk

Although South Asians are not a uniform group, and the prevalence of traditional cardiovascular risk factors may vary between the various sub-groups, the fact remains that in virtually every study reported in South Asians, the risks of type 2 diabetes and CVD are magnified compared with white European populations.[1–8] In addition, it is clear that the classical risk factors do not fully explain the increased risk in this population, since risk prediction models such as Framingham and SCORE tend to underestimate CHD risk by approximately 50%.

There is evidence that South Asians have an increased propensity to develop the metabolic syndrome compared with other populations as described by Cappuccio in chapter 3. The syndrome appears to relate to insulin resistance as a central feature (resistance of the body to the biological actions of insulin) and describes a co-occurrence of major cardiovascular risk factors in the same person.[11, 12] There is now good evidence that this syndrome, which includes a strong tendency to abdominal (central) obesity, is more common in UK South Asians and may account, at least in part, for the excess cardiovascular risk.[2, 10]

It is likely that there is a common mechanism which links the increased prevalence of both type 2 diabetes and CVD in this population. The major arbiters of insulin resistance are obesity (particularly abdominal/central obesity) and sedentary lifestyle, although genetic factors are also likely to be involved. As long ago as the 1960s, the geneticist Neel postulated the 'thrifty genotype' hypothesis.[13] He suggested that during the course of evolution, people who possessed genes which enabled them to lay down fat stores during times of food abundance would have a survival advantage in times of famine. This survival advantage has now become a liability in populations where there are now 'continuous times of plenty'! It is likely that certain populations, and this includes the South Asian population, have an increased genetic susceptibility to lay down intra-abdominal fat, particularly when they meet a Western style of living. Migration and urbanisation have led to significant changes in dietary patterns over a short period of time (high sugar, high fat type of diet) which the body can no longer cope with largely due to a sedentary lifestyle.

There is evidence that the UK South Asian population has a more sedentary lifestyle than the corresponding white European population[3, 14] and they also have a tendency to increased insulin resistance.[2, 15–16] Insulin resistance is associated with hyperinsulinaemia (the body's 'attempt' to overcome insulin resistance) and this in turn predisposes to a dyslipidaemic lipid profile and an increase in low density lipoproteins (LDL) and very low density lipoproteins (VLDL) and reduction in high density lipoproteins (HDL).[1, 12] This is a highly atherogenic risk profile. There is also evidence that hyperinsulinaemia is associated with increased risk of hypertension, perhaps in part because of increased sodium re-absorption from the proximal renal tubule and increased sympathetic nervous system stimulation.[17, 18] In a proportion of people with the metabolic syndrome, the pancreas is unable to produce sufficient insulin to overcome the insulin resistance with development of relative insulin deficiency, followed by impaired glucose tolerance and frank type 2 diabetes.[11, 12]

It is important to stress that accepted criteria for metabolic syndrome do not necessarily require a diagnosis of type 2 diabetes to be made. The NCEP ATPIII Guidelines[19] suggest that the metabolic syndrome can be defined on the basis of at least three of five major risk factors i.e.

- increased waist circumference (a very good surrogate marker for intra-abdominal fat) >102 cm in men, >88 cm in women
- reduced HDL cholesterol (<1.1 mmol/l men and <1.3 mmol/l women)
- increased triglycerides (>1.7 mmol/l)
- hypertension (BP ≥ 130/85) and
- a fasting blood glucose >6.1 mmol/l (6.1–6.9 mmol/l is defined as impaired fasting glucose and ≥7 mmol as type 2 diabetes).

The result is that most patients with type 2 diabetes do indeed suffer from the metabolic syndrome but the converse is also true i.e. most people with metabolic syndrome do not suffer from diabetes! Having said this, many of them will have some evidence of dysglycaemia if sophisticated tests are done.

The average BMI of the South Asian population in the UK is not greater than that of the corresponding white European population. South Asians do, however, have a much greater tendency to lay down intra-abdominal fat which is metabolically active and is strongly related to insulin resistance.[20–22] The realisation that South Asians tend to suffer the consequences of being overweight at a much lower level than the white European population has led the World Health Organisation (WHO) to recently recommend the redefinition of obesity in the South Asian population as BMI >25 kg/m^2 (obesity in white Europeans still defined at BMI >30 kg/m^2) and that overweight is BMI >23 kg/m^2 (rather than >25 kg/m^2 in white Europeans).[23] There has also been increased emphasis on abdominal circumference as an even better marker for risk of type 2 diabetes, CVD and metabolic syndrome, than BMI and many believe it should be measured as a standard risk marker as part of the new General Practitioner Contract (GMS2) in the UK. Measurement of waist circumference is now a necessary part of standard definitions/diagnoses of metabolic syndrome (including the recent International Diabetes Federation recommendation as shown in Table 3.1).

Comparison of cardiovascular risk factors in South Asians and white Europeans living in the UK

Several studies have suggested that the excess risk for cardiovascular mortality in the South Asian population cannot be entirely explained by their high prevalence of glucose intolerance.[8, 24] There is some evidence, however, that diabetes disproportionately increases CHD mortality in UK South Asians.[24] As already stated, average BMI is also not greater in UK Asians and white Europeans but the former tend to be much more seriously affected by the consequences of being overweight.

Several studies have not shown a significant difference in blood pressure values between the various populations compared with white Europeans[3,8] although in one study in South London it was found that the UK South Asians of both sexes have a higher prevalence of hypertension than white Europeans.[25] Rates of smoking also do not differ significantly between South Asians and white Europeans in the UK and in fact rates of smoking amongst South Asian females are very low. Reduced physical activity has been demonstrated in UK Asians compared with white Europeans and may reflect the increased tendency to insulin resistance and type 2 diabetes.[3, 14] Various other risk markers, including concentrations of fibrinogen and plasminogen activator inhibitor 1

(PAI-1) have been studied and found to be increased in South Asians compared to white Europeans[26] and, similarly, impaired endothelial function and raised CRP have been found more commonly in UK South Asians compared with white Europeans.[27–29]

Perhaps the most striking difference is in the lipid profiles of the two groups, although not all studies have confirmed this. Important features defining the metabolic syndrome include low HDL cholesterol and raised triglycerides (TG) and this is an atherogenic profile.[11] Several studies have shown this pattern more commonly in South Asian populations than white Europeans,[14, 30, 31] although South Asian people do not have higher total LDL cholesterol. It is likely that, as with overweight/obesity, South Asians are more adversely affected at lower thresholds of dyslipidaemia compared with white European populations.

It is interesting to note that although total plasma cholesterol may actually be lower in UK South Asians than white Europeans, it is still significantly higher than that seen in South Asians in India.[32] Migration has been clearly shown to be associated with increased cholesterol levels in this population[32] and they also appear to have an increased serum lipoprotein (a) concentration (Lp(a)) which is genetically determined.[32, 33] Lp(a) has been shown to be an independent risk factor for early atherosclerosis and the effect is magnified where LDL or total cholesterol to HDL ratio is increased.[30, 33]

One study, which looked at coronary risk factors in migrants from the Punjab living in West London compared to their siblings still living in the Punjab, clearly demonstrated much higher prevalence of coronary risk factors in the migrants.[32] These included higher total cholesterol, BMI, systolic blood pressure, apolipoprotein B and fasting blood glucose. This was accompanied by lower HDL and increased insulin resistance and beta cell dysfunction compared with siblings in the Punjab. Lp(a) was similar in the two groups but higher than in white Europeans.

All these data support the idea that for a given level of risk factor, South Asians are potentially more seriously affected by atheroma formation than the white European population. This is particularly pertinent for the lipid profile where typically many South Asians have low HDL cholesterol, raised triglycerides, high serum LDL and high serum Lp(a) concentrations. This is proposed as an explanation for the 'malignant' atherosclerosis commonly seen in relatively young South Asians.[30] It is also clear that raised total or LDL cholesterol remain important risk factors for development of coronary artery disease in UK Asians just as they do in white Europeans. The consequences of an increase in total or LDL cholesterol in South Asians may be proportionally greater than in white European populations for reasons that are not clear. Looking specifically at triglycerides, these are almost always higher in studies in South Asians compared with white Europeans.[14, 30, 31] This is so even when levels of physical activity are taken into account. The same applies for HDL where the majority of studies have reported HDL levels lower in UK Asians compared with white Europeans. The typical dyslipidaemia of diabetes includes raised TG and reduced HDL cholesterol (part of the metabolic syndrome) and it is interesting that the dyslipidaemia seen in UK South Asians generally reflects this pattern more. This emphasises the point again that South Asians are more likely to have the metabolic syndrome and evidence of dysglycaemia.

Evidence base for treatment

There is no particular reason to suppose that the evidence that we have largely from white European populations for cardiovascular protection would also not apply to the South Asian population. Indeed, all would agree that a 'healthy eating' type of diet and increased physical activity, together with stopping cigarette smoking, should be encouraged. There is little doubt also that strict control of blood pressure and lipids, and perhaps addition of low dose aspirin, are a sensible form of management.

There are, though, a number of important points to emphasise. Most importantly, and as already described, South Asians living in the UK tend to get heart disease earlier and perhaps have a worse prognosis long term than their white European counterparts. They also have a much higher risk of development of type 2 diabetes possibly related to metabolic syndrome abnormalities. Certainly, as already discussed, SMR data are much higher than for the general population and this may relate to diabetes and CVD. A number of studies have demonstrated that moderate to high physical activity significantly reduces the risk of CHD, and physical activity levels are generally low in UK Asians.[14, 33] The energy intake as fat in UK South Asians is comparable to that in white Europeans but is double that of non-migrant Indian Asians. Encouragement to reduce fat intake is sensible, therefore, and particularly to avoid the use of ghee which is used in home cooking and known to be atherogenic.[34]

The evidence base for treatment of people at high cardiovascular risk with statins is now so profound that one really needs to ask why one would NOT use a statin in a particular patient, rather than whether one should. This is particularly the case in South Asian diabetic patients. Indeed, studies have demonstrated that type 2 diabetes is a cardiovascular risk equivalent[35] and many now argue, based on recent publication of the Heart Protection Study (HPS)[36] (Figure 6.2) and the CARDS study[37] (Figure 6.3), that all type 2 diabetic patients should be prescribed a statin.

The National Institute for Clinical Excellence (NICE) has recommended that all diabetic patients with a 10-year CHD risk >15% be prescribed a statin.[38] This equates to around 70% of all diabetic patients with the remaining 30% usually not reaching this threshold level purely because of youth! One might then ask the question – why wait another 10 years until they reach the 15% risk threshold as this may allow 10 years of atheroma formation? This is particularly the case in South Asian diabetic patients who commonly

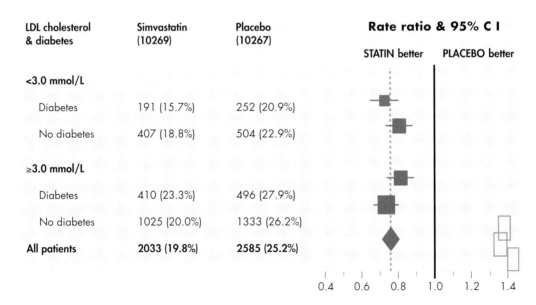

Figure 6.2 Heart Protection Study (HPS) demonstrating significant reduction in cardiovascular endpoints and mortality with statin usage in diabetic patients. ADAPTED FROM REF 36 AND REPRINTED WITH PERMISSION FROM ELSEVIER (ON BEHALF OF THE LANCET)

develop diabetes at a much younger age, plus the fact that they are in any case at greatly increased cardiovascular risk compared with the white European population. **It is our opinion that all type 2 diabetic patients should normally be prescribed a statin unless there is a contraindication or tolerability problem. This applies doubly to South Asian diabetics! In our view, risk tables are redundant in guiding pharmacotherapeutic intervention in diabetes – all diabetic patients should be treated from the point of view of secondary prevention.**

The above argument may also apply to low dose aspirin. The evidence base for aspirin usage is not as good as with statins, but the Hypertension Optimal Treatment (HOT) study demonstrated a 15% risk reduction for cardiovascular end points in diabetic patients treated with low dose aspirin, albeit with increased risk of (non-fatal) haemorrhage.[39] In our clinic, we normally prescribe low dose aspirin (75mg) once blood pressure is controlled (systolic <150 mm/Hg) in all diabetic patients over the age of 50 years and in those under 50 years if there is a history of CVD or they have at least one other cardiovascular risk factor (unless there is a contraindication or tolerability problem).

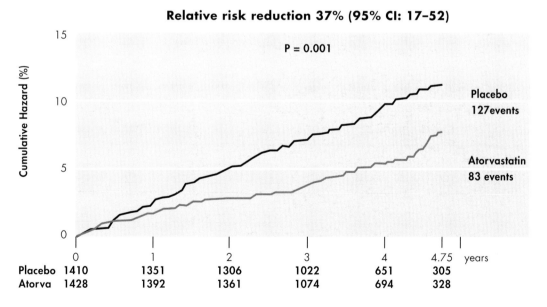

Figure 6.3 CARDS study demonstrating significant reduction in cardiovascular endpoints and mortality with statin usage in diabetic patients ADAPTED FROM REF 37 AND REPRINTED WITH PERMISSION FROM ELSEVIER (ON BEHALF OF THE LANCET)

It is also apparent that recommendations arising from, for example, the GMS2 Contract for GPs put the cholesterol target at too high a level. All the evidence we have is that 'the lower the better'. The GMS Contract target of total cholesterol of 5mmol/l is now significantly higher than recent guidelines from the USA and Europe which suggest a target for total cholesterol and LDL cholesterol of 4.5 or even 4mmol/l and 2.5 or even 2.0mmol/l respectively. Where statins alone do not get down to target LDL, a cholesterol absorption inhibitor (ezetimibe) can also be considered in combination with a statin.

Although there is an excellent evidence base for reduction in cardiovascular morbidity and mortality by use of statins in high cardiovascular risk populations, it should be remembered that the typical dyslipidaemia of metabolic syndrome is not so much an increase in LDL or total cholesterol but more a tendency to low HDL and raised TG. There is good evidence that low HDL is associated with increased cardiovascular risk and that one of the best markers of such risk is total cholesterol to HDL ratio. The evidence for TG being an independent risk factor for CVD is less robust but certainly plausible. It follows from this that South Asians with type 2 diabetes should all be on a statin unless there are tolerability or contraindication type problems. It also follows that non-diabetic South Asians should also be on a statin if they are at sufficiently high cardiovascular risk (and that to estimate risk from a primary prevention point of view, 50% should be added to the value obtained using standard risk tables).

For patients with type 2 diabetes who are prescribed a statin, should an agent which causes a rise in HDL also be prescribed where the latter is reduced? It certainly seems logical in this situation to prescribe a statin with a fibrate or nicotinic acid derivative, although the evidence base for such an approach is certainly much less robust than for statin prescribing. It should also be remembered that use of a combination of statin plus fibrate, for example, is associated with an increased risk of side-effects. It would, though, seem reasonable to prescribe such a combination with a statin where HDL is significantly reduced e.g. <1mmol/l in high risk individuals. Clearly, if TG are very high (say above 8mmol/l) then a fibrate becomes mandatory to at least reduce the risk of development of acute pancreatitis if not that of CVD.

Cultural issues

There are clearly significant issues which include a range of problems which may arise from inability to speak or read English (particularly in older Asian females), lifestyle differences and deprivation. It is also clear that many South Asians are not using health resources adequately and we and others have shown that South Asians are less likely to be prescribed statins and other cardioprotective treatments.[40, 41] This is despite a higher CHD morbidity and mortality compared with white Europeans. Clearly, preventative treatment strategies need to be tailored to the needs of individual ethnic groups, taking into consideration both cultural acceptability as well as increased risk. There is an urgent need to increase awareness of diabetes and CVD in these populations and also the measures that can be taken to reduce risk.

The above will require the help of health professionals but also population-based strategies to promote important messages to help preserve health, including reduction in insulin resistance through weight loss and increased physical activity. Differences in cooking methods need to be taken into account, as well as a host of other cultural and language difficulties.

Summary

South Asians living in the UK have an increased risk of both type 2 diabetes and CHD compared with the white European population. There is a whole range of reasons for this, both genetic and environmental. South Asians appear to have increased susceptibility to development of insulin resistance when they meet certain environmental factors which include being overweight and adoption of a sedentary lifestyle. This may relate to an increased tendency to lay down abdominal fat, which is metabolically active and strongly related to development of insulin resistance. This appears to be a central feature of the metabolic syndrome with consequent increased risk of CVD and type 2 diabetes. South Asians have a 4–6 fold increased prevalence of type 2 diabetes compared with the white European population and it tends to occur at a younger age with commonly more devastating consequences.

Approaches to the problem need to be at both the population and individual level. Clearly, more resource needs to be put into education, including health awareness campaigns, encouragement of healthy lifestyle and aggressive management where required. At an individual level, we now have an excellent evidence base for treatment of vascular risk factors such as dyslipidaemia, hypertension and hyperglycaemia. It is clear, though, that this evidence is not being comprehensively applied across the population group and that there is a massive degree of under-treatment of these risk factors. It is also clear that risk tables do not take into account ethnicity or indeed, for diabetic patients, degree of diabetic control and presence of microalbuminuria. Certainly, in the South Asian population they grossly underestimate risk. If conventional risk tables are to be used in South Asian people in the UK then 50% needs to be added to the calculated value for cardiovascular risk to take into account the excess risk. It is our opinion that risk tables should not be used at all in patients with type 2 diabetes except for research or descriptive purposes; i.e. we should think of type 2 diabetes as a CVD and therefore appropriate for secondary prevention. This is particularly the case in South Asian patients.

It is also clear that, in many cases, South Asians are not getting as comprehensive healthcare as white European people and there may be a host of reasons for this including cultural and communication difficulties. For these reasons, new approaches to management need to be developed which take into account these issues with the long-term aim of reducing morbidity and mortality from diabetes and CVD in this patient group. It is this awareness that led to the setting up of the United Kingdom Asian Diabetes Study (UKADS) which will be described in the next part of this paper.

The United Kingdom Asian Diabetes Study (UKADS)

This is a culturally sensitive, community-based, multiple cardiovascular risk factor intervention study comparing outcomes versus standard care in practices provided with enhanced Practice Nurse time, Asian Linkworkers and community-based Diabetes Specialist Nurses working to specific algorithms for blood pressure, lipid and glycaemic control.[41] The results of the pilot phase of the study have been recently published and will be described and reviewed briefly, followed by description of a much larger study which has recently started.

The UKADS – pilot data

In addition to the increased risk of type 2 diabetes and excess cardiovascular mortality in South Asians, they also tend to have a higher prevalence of microalbuminuria and later development of renal complications.[42,43] The problem is further magnified by cultural and communication difficulties, together with background deprivation in some communities.

The United Kingdom Prospective Diabetes Study (UKPDS)[44,45] has already established the effectiveness of tight glycaemic and blood pressure control and there is also now a wealth of evidence that use of statins in high risk individuals is associated with dramatic reductions in cardiovascular risk. In the UKADS, we ask the question whether there is a cost-effective and acceptable way to translate UKPDS and lipid findings in South Asians. We hypothesize that the introduction of structured, culturally sensitive care for diabetes in the South Asian community can improve cardiovascular risk factors and ultimately cardiovascular endpoints in a cost-effective manner. This is to be achieved by Asian Linkworkers, community Diabetes Specialist Nurses and Practice Nurses working to joint protocols with clearly defined targets.

The aims of the pilot were to determine whether this approach (compared with standard care) was associated with improvement in blood pressure, lipids and glycaemic control with the eventual aim of reducing both microvascular progression and cardiovascular endpoints. A further aim was to measure cost and compare cost and short-term outcomes with current practice. We planned, if the pilot results justified this, to produce a generalisable risk reduction strategy for the management of type 2 diabetes in South Asian patients which could be evaluated in a large-scale trial.

Six general practices from Birmingham and Coventry were randomised – three to receive the intervention and three conventional care. We used simple algorithms to attempt to reduce vascular risk by strict control of blood pressure, lipids and glycaemia. The algorithms were made available to all practices but in the active intervention group the protocols were implemented by community-based Diabetes Nurse Educators working with Practice Nurses. The Practice Nurses were provided with enhanced time and supported by Asian Linkworkers who also worked with community pharmacists and community leaders in implementation of protocols and to enhance treatment compliance.

In the pilot phase of the study we recruited 401 patients, half intervention, half control. A range of measurements were made, including blood pressure, lipid profile, HbA_{1c}, BMI, waist circumference and albumin/creatinine ratios. The mean age of participants at baseline was 59 years with a mean duration of diabetes of 8 years but with very wide distribution. Around 70% of patients were on oral hypoglycaemic agents, 14% on diet alone and 16% on insulin $\pm$ oral hypoglycaemic agents. Thirteen percent of the cohort were current smokers (almost all men – i.e. around 25% of males were current smokers and very few females). Current alcohol consumption was around 13% (again, mostly males i.e. around 25% of males).

Based on the new WHO definition of obesity already described, 95% of the patients were overweight (BMI >23 kg/m^2) and 80% of them were obese (BMI >25 kg/m^2). Indeed, 45% were grossly obese with BMIs >30 kg/m^2. At baseline just over half the patients had systolic blood pressure above 140 and diastolic blood pressure above 80 mmHg, with mean blood pressure 145/82 mmHg and a very wide distribution of blood pressures across the group. From the point of view of baseline data, there was an extremely interesting relationship with systolic blood pressure and albumin excretion rate. Although it was true that both micro- and macroalbuminuria increased with increasing blood pressure, even in those patients with normotension around one third had micro- or macroproteinuria. This is considerably higher than in white European patients.

In addition, 58% of patients had a total cholesterol >5 mmol/l (mean 5.3 $\pm$ 1.2 mmol/l), and two thirds of patients had an HbA_{1c} >7% (mean 8 $\pm$ 2%). There was no significant difference between the two groups from the point of view of sex, age, duration of diabetes, treatment, smoking, alcohol consumption, blood pressure, total cholesterol or HbA_{1c}.

After one year of follow-up (Table 6.1), there was a significantly greater fall in mean systolic blood pressure in the intervention group compared with the control group. This was also seen for diastolic blood pressure and total cholesterol. There was no significant difference in HbA_{1c} between the groups.

This pilot study helped to produce an infrastructure with the right partnerships, and further development of protocols and educational tools. It confirmed the feasibility of

Table 6.1 Risk factor change over 1 year of follow up					
	Intervention Mean Difference	Control Mean Difference	Difference	95% CI	P value
Systolic BP	-6.69	-2.11	-4.58	-8.84 to -0.32	0.035
Diastolic BP	-3.14	+0.28	-3.14	-5.66 to -1.16	0.003
Total cholesterol	-0.51	-0.12	-0.38	-0.65 to +0.12	0.005
HbA_{1c}	-0.23	-0.20	-0.03	-0.36 to +0.30	0.866

applying this strategy in primary care involving 400 patients. It also produced important insights into the nature and prevalence of complications, cardiovascular risk and obesity in the South Asian group and we demonstrated reduction in important cardiovascular risk factors, i.e. blood pressure and lipids, in the 'active' practices.

The question remains as to whether this approach can produce sustained results over time in a larger population. Full health economic evaluation also needs to be performed; there is not much point in improving cardiovascular risk if the cost breaks the health economy! It might also be important to look at the practical ways of enacting the various protocols/algorithms, including examining the feasibility of nurse prescribing through patient group directives for cardiovascular risk factors and incorporation of 'expert patient' led education sessions. It will also be important to include quantitative studies to examine reasons for the inability to achieve targets by control practices and to determine what works within active practices. A white European diabetic control group would also be very useful, at least to give some background information.

UKADS – the major study

The relative success of the pilot study has encouraged us to proceed with a much larger study along the lines suggested above. The recruitment phase is now finished, with 18 practices from Birmingham and Coventry each recruiting around 100 South Asian diabetic patients for this study. The larger study is based on a cluster randomisation of practices into 'active' and 'control/conventional' care. Several of the conventional care practices are also recruiting 500 white European diabetic patients to give background information. The study is planned to run for 3 years after randomisation with a recording of cardiovascular risk markers and major outcomes.

The protocol is similar to that for the pilot with nurse-led delivery and protected Practice Nurse time. The Practice Nurses are trained by the UKADS community-based Nurse Coordinator and they run intensive control clinics monthly until targets are met. Asian Linkworkers help find and educate high risk patients with strong collaboration with community Diabetes Specialist Nurses and the Practice Nurse.

Importantly, all the practices are provided with the same management guidelines, with similar algorithms to those described above. Several changes, though, have been made to the guidelines/algorithms to take into account the much tighter blood pressure and lipid targets currently recommended by various national and international bodies. This has led to a blood pressure target of <130/80 mmHg (recent British Hypertension Society guidelines) and total cholesterol <4 mmol/l (various national and international guidelines). In addition, given that there was no significant improvement in HbA_{1c} in either group in the pilot, the glycaemic control algorithm has been tightened to allow for much more rapid and aggressive intervention. The community-based Diabetes Specialist Nurse supports target attainment and audits conventional care clinics. We had planned to allow nurse prescribing in active practices but this has so far not been enacted due to logistic reasons.

We plan to compare active versus conventional practices with regard to the proportion achieving target values, as well as absolute reductions in risk factors. This will include patient satisfaction and quality of life questionnaires. Outcomes will include cardiovascular risk analysis with measurement of blood pressure and lipids, HbA_{1c}, BMI, waist circumference, plasma creatinine, albumin/creatinine ratio, ECG, diabetes knowledge and quality of life. Major outcomes will also be recorded, including hospital admissions and referrals. Death, myocardial infarction, stroke, amputation, blindness and retinal laser treatment will also be recorded. A sub-group will be analysed from the point of view of retinal photography.

Importantly, economic evaluation is seen as a major part of this project. We will measure intervention and treatment costs, and compare costs and consequences. This will involve decision modelling analysis in order to model costs and benefits. This will be done through collaborations with the University of Warwick Business School. This data will provide an analysis for Primary Care Trusts and the Strategic Health Authority as well as clinicians.

To date, all of the South Asian patients have been enrolled and we will soon also complete enrolment of white European subjects with type 2 diabetes. All subjects have been requested also to provide blood for DNA extraction for genetic analysis so that we presently also have a very large, well characterised database for such studies. We have DNA from South Asian subjects with type 2 diabetes, South Asian non-diabetic controls and white European subjects with type 2 diabetes. We have available a great deal of clinical information on these subjects and the database is sufficiently large to allow some division of subjects according to racial origin. Our initial work involved studies of the genetics of dyslipidaemia in these populations, although a range of other candidate genes are also planned for study. This type of work will provide invaluable data for this population who are at such high diabetes and cardiovascular risk.

Conclusion

The prevalence of both type 2 diabetes and CVD is dramatically magnified in the South Asian population in the UK (and many other countries) compared with the indigenous white European population. These problems occur commonly at a younger age and there is some evidence that this in part relates to abdominal central/visceral adiposity and insulin resistance. South Asians are more likely to have an atherogenic dyslipidaemia consisting of low HDL and raised triglycerides. There is also evidence that there is significant under-treatment in this patient group for a whole host of reasons.

The UKADS pilot has demonstrated that a structured, culturally sensitive, community-based approach to cardiovascular risk management can be successful in a type 2 diabetic population of South Asian extraction. It remains to be seen whether such an approach can be equally applied in a cost-effective manner in a similar but much larger population.

Failure to enact comprehensively the evidence base already available for cardiovascular risk reduction in the South Asian population will doom many people from this community to an early death from type 2 diabetes and CVD.

Acknowledgements

We would like to acknowledge the help and support of all general practitioners, their practice nurses and other health care workers involved in the UKADS study. We would also like to thank the UKADS Executive Committee for all their help and advice – these include JP O'Hare, NT Raymond, S Mughal, L Dodd, W Hanif, Y Ahmad, K Mishra, A Jones, S Kumar, A Szczepura and EW Hillhouse.

We would also like to thank the following companies for providing financial support in the form of grants for the UKADS: Pfizer, Aventis UK, Servier Labs UK, MSD/Schering-Plough, Takeda UK, Roche, Boehringer Ingelheim, Eli Lilly, Novo Nordisk, Bristol Myers Squibb, Sankyo, Merck and Sanofi-Synthelabo.

This paper is based on a lecture given by AH Barnett at the South Asian Health Foundation meeting held in Oxford, UK, in December 2004.

References

1. Dept of Health National Service Framework for Diabetes: Standards. 2001/2.

2. Knight TM, Smith Z, Whittles A, Sahota P, Locton JA, Hogg G et al. Insulin resistance, diabetes, and risk markers for ischaemic heart disease in Asian men and non-Asians in Bradford. *Br Heart J* 1992; **67**: 343–50.

3. McKeigue PM, Ferrie J, Pierpoint T, Marmot MG. Association of early-onset coronary heart disease in South Asian men with glucose intolerance and hyperinsulinaemia. *Circulation* 1993; **87**: 152–61.

4. Cappuccio FP, Cook DG, Atkinson RW, Wicks PD. The Wandsworth Heart and Stroke Study. A population-based survey of cardiovascular risk factor in different ethnic groups. Methods and baseline findings. *Nutr Metab Cardiovasc Dis* 1998; **8**: 371–85.

5. NHS National Service Framework for Coronary Artery Disease 2000.

6. Wild S, McKeigue P. Cross sectional analysis of mortality by country of birth in England and Wales, 1970–92. *Br Med J* 1997; **314**: 705.

7. Balarajan R. Ethnic differences in mortality from ischaemic heart disease and cerebrovascular disease in England and Wales. *Br Med J* 1991; **302**: 560–4.

8. McKeigue PM, Miller GJ, Marmot MG. Coronary heart disease in South Asians overseas – review. *J Clin Epidemiol* 1989; **422**: 597–609.

9. Hughes LO, Raval U, Raftery EB. First myocardial infarctions in Asian and white men. *Br Med J* 1989; **298**: 1345–50.

10. Gupta S, de Belder A, Hughes LO. Avoiding premature coronary deaths in Asians in Britain. *Br Med J* 1995; **311**: 1035–1036.

11. Reaven GM. Banting lecture 1988. Role of insulin resistance in human disease. *Diabetes* 1988; **37**(12): 1595–1607.

12. Barnett AH and O'Gara G. *Diabetes and CVD*. London: MEP Ltd 2004.

13. Neel JV. Diabetes mellitus: a 'thrifty' genotype rendered detrimental by 'progress'? *Am J Hum Genet* 1962; **14**: 353–362.

14. Bhopal R, Unwin N, White M, Yallop J, Walker L, Alberti KGMM et al. Heterogeneity of coronary heart disease risk factors in Indian, Pakistani, Bangladeshi, and European origin populations: cross sectional study. *Br Med J* 1999; **19**: 215–20.

15. McKeigue PM, Marmot MG. Mortality from coronary heart disease in Asian communities in London. *Br Med J* 1988; **297**: 903.

16. McKeigue PM, Shah B, Marmot MG. Relation of central obesity and insulin resistance with high diabetes prevalence and cardiovascular risk in South Asians. *Lancet* 1991; **337**: 382–6.

17. DeFronzo RA. The effect of insulin on renal sodium metabolism. A review with clinical implications. *Diabetologia* 1981; **21**: 165–171.

18. Rowe JW, Young JB, Minaker KL et al. Effect of insulin and glucose infusions on sympathetic nervous system activity in normal man. *Diabetes* 1981; **30**: 219–225.

19. National Cholesterol Education Program. Third Report of the Expert Panel on Detection, Evaluation, and Treatment of High Blood Cholesterol in Adults (Adult Treatment Panel III). Bethesda, MD: National Institute of Health 2002.

20. Jensen MD, Haymond MW, Rizza RA et al. Influence of body fat distribution on free fatty acid metabolism in obesity. *J Clin Invest* 1989; **83**(4): 1168–1173.

21. McTernan P, Kumar S. Pathogenesis of obesity-related type 2 diabetes. In: Barnett AH, Kumar S (eds). *Obesity and Diabetes: Wiley Diabetes in Practice Series*. Chichester: John Wiley & Sons 2004; 49–78.

22. Steppan CM, Bailey ST, Bhat S et al. The hormone resistin links obesity to diabetes. *Nature* 2001; **409**: 307–312.

23. International Diabetes Institute (World Health Organization). Co-sponsored by the Regional Office for the Western Pacific, WHO, International Association for the Study of Obesity and the International Obesity Task Force. *The Asia-Pacific Perspective: redefining obesity and its treatment*. Sydney: Health Communications Australia 2000.

24. Chaturvedi N, Fuller JH. Ethnic differences in mortality from CVD in the UK: do they persist in people with diabetes? *J Epidemiol Community Health* 1996; **50**: 137–9.

25. Cappuccio FP, Cook DG, Atkinson RW, Strazzullo P. Prevalence, detection, and management of cardiovascular risk factors in different ethnic groups in south London. *Heart* 1997; **78**: 555–63.

26. Kain K, Catto AJ, Grant PJ. Impaired finrinolysis and increased fibrinogen levels in South Asian subjects. *Atherosclerosis* 2001; **156**: 457–61.

27. Chambers JC, McGregor A, Jean-Marie J, Kooner JS. Abnormalities of vascular endothelial function may contribute to increased coronary heart disease risk in UK Indian Asians. *Heart* 1999; **81**: 501–4.

28. Chambers JC, Obeid OA, Refsum H, Ueland P, Hackett D, Hooper J et al. Plasma homocysteine concentrations and risk of coronary heart disease in UK Indian Asian and European men. *Lancet* 2000; **355**: 523–27.

29. Chambers JC, Eda S, Bassett P, Karim Y, Thompson SG, Gallimore JR et al. C-Reactive protein, insulin resistance, central obesity, and coronary heart disease risk in Indian Asians from the United Kingdom compared with European Whites. *Circulation* 2001; **104**: 145–150.

30. Enas EA, Mehta J. Malignant coronary artery disease in young Asian Indians: thoughts on pathogenesis, prevention, and therapy. Coronary Artery Disease in Asian Indians (CADI) Study. *Clin Cardiol* 1995; **18**: 131–5.

31. Whitty CJM, Brunner EJ, Shipley MJ, Hemingway H, Marmot MG. Differences in biological risk factors for CVD between three ethnic groups in the Whitehall study. *Atherosclerosis* 1999; **142**: 279–86.

32. Bhatnagar D, Anand IS, Durrington PN, Patel DJ, Wander GS, Mackness MI et al. Coronary risk factors in people from the Indian subcontinent living in West London and their siblings in India. *Lancet* 1995; **345**: 405–9.

33. Cardiovascular disorders. Primary prevention. *Clinical Evidence* 2003: 133–152.

34. Kooner JS. Coronary heart disease in UK Asians: the potential for reducing mortality. *Heart* 1997; **78**: 530–2.

35. Haffner SM, Lehto S, Ronnemaa T et al. Mortality from coronary heart disease in subjects with type 2 diabetes and in non-diabetic subjects with and without prior myocardial infarction. *N Engl J Med* 1998; **339**: 229–234.

36. Heart Protection Study Collaborative Group. MRC/BHF Heart Protection Study of cholesterol lowering with simvastatin in 20,536 high-risk individuals: a randomised placebo-controlled trial. *Lancet* 2002; **360**: 7–22.

37. Colhoun HM, Betteridge DJ, Durrington PN et al. Primary prevention of CVD with atorvastatin in type 2 diabetes in the Collaborative Atorvastatin Diabetes Study (CARDS): multicentre randomised placebo-controlled trial. *Lancet* 2004; **364**: 685–696.

38. National Institute for Clinical Excellence. *Management of type 2 diabetes – management of blood pressure and blood lipids* (Guideline H). London: NICE 2002 (www.nice.org.uk).

39. Hansson L, Zanchetti A, Carruthers SG et al. Effects of intensive blood-pressure lowering and low-dose aspirin in patients with hypertension: principal results of the Hypertension Optimal Treatment (HOT) randomised trial. HOT Study Group. *Lancet* 1998; **351**: 1755–1762.

40. Patel MG, Wright DJ, Gill PS, Jerwood D, Silcok J, Chrystyn H. Prescribing of lipid lowering drugs to South Asian patients: ecological study. *Br Med J* 2002; **325**: 25–6.

41. O'Hare JP, Raymond NT, Mughal S et al. Evaluation of delivery of enhanced diabetes care to patients of South Asian ethnicity: the United Kingdom Asian Diabetes Study (UKADS). *Diabetic Medicine*; **21**: 1357–1365.

42. Raleigh VS, Kim V, Balarajan R. Variations in mortality from diabetes mellitus, hypertension and renal disease in England and Wales by country of birth. *Health Trends* 1997; **28**: 122–127.

43. Balarajan R. Ethnicity and variations in mortality from coronary heart disease. *Health Trends* 1996; **28**: 45–51.

44. UK Prospective Diabetes Study Group. Intensive blood glucose control with sulphonylureas or insulin compared with conventional treatment and risk of complications in patients with type 2 diabetes (UKPDS33). *Lancet* 1998; **352**: 837–853.

45. UK Prospective Diabetes Study Group. Tight blood pressure control and risk of macrovascular and microvascular complication in type 2 diabetes (UKPDS38). *Br Med J* 1998; **317**: 703–713.

7
Mobilising communities: the Khush Dil experience

Gill Mathews

Introduction

The higher incidence of diabetes, stroke and Coronary Heart Disease (CHD) in people of South Asian origin living in the UK carries significant consequences for the health of local populations and for NHS resources.[1] Previous chapters have explored the reasons for this anomaly in depth. Suffice to say here that the increased incidence is acknowledged as complex and multifaceted in nature, refusing to be solely explained by the existence of typical CHD risk markers.[2, 3] Coupled with difficulties with access to health care services, research findings highlight genetic differences, lower socio-economic status and racism as additional important factors.[3–7]

To help address this plethora of inequality, NHS policymakers have highlighted the need for health service providers to become more responsive to the lifestyles and cultures of different minority ethnic groups.[6,7] The Race Relations (Amendment) Act 2000 imposed a duty on all public bodies to promote equality of opportunity and good race relations[8] and Fair for All (2001) set out a framework for action to address equality and diversity issues. Within this improved delivery of health services to black and minority ethnic (BME) communities is advocated including recommendations for targeted action on chronic disease management where morbidity is high.[7] As a localised response, Khush Dil, an Edinburgh-based community health project, was set up following consultations with South Asian people about health needs. The project focused on how primary care staff might better raise awareness in communities about the higher prevalence of CHD and diabetes, and what could be done to improve access to prevention services.

The main aim of Khush Dil was to run as a primary prevention pilot developing a culturally appropriate framework for the identification, screening and management of CHD risk factors. It was surmised that this could then become incorporated within primary care mainstream provision. Service delivery revolved around community outreach screening and dietetic clinics supported by a programme of healthy lifestyle activities. This chapter summarises Khush Dil activities, its clinical impact on the health of participants, and key learning from the project highlighting the challenges ahead in respect of mainstreaming.

Project outline

Community development principles underpinned the framework for service planning and delivery, embracing multi-disciplinary working, cross-sectoral partnership, public participation and outreach. Close liaison with the voluntary sector and minority ethnic workers was essential to run effective grass roots health promotion programmes. These incorporated clinical screening as one dimension of a series of activities and workshops designed to raise awareness and provide practical support to address coronary risk factors. South Asian community workers were particularly important, acting as cultural advisers to the small staff team, networking with local people and, vitally, raising awareness about CHD risk through health promotion work.

Primary to Khush Dil were the following service elements:

- Health-visitor-led screening to identify and address coronary risk factors
- Dietetic clinics to provide 1:1 nutritional support
- Practical activities to encourage lifestyle change and reduce CHD risk including cookery workshops, exercise classes and CHD/diabetes awareness sessions.

Activities

Healthy heart/dietetic clinics

Time-intensive screening and dietetic clinics were run from the project base and various community venues including local religious bases, voluntary organisations and restaurants with interpretation and translation supplied via the local council service or South Asian health workers.

1:1 cardiac health assessment was carried out using a validated coronary risk assessment package.[9] Computer graphics gave the patient a visual picture of their individual heart health profile, identifying any CHD risk factors and denoting levels of risk in bar chart form. This chart was then used as a platform for discussion of risk factors with the graphics providing a user-friendly way of promoting awareness about CHD risk and a clear focus for motivational interviewing and individual goal-setting.

Each person's stage of change was assessed in relation to their motivation to address lifestyle behaviours overall using working definitions derived from the literature on the transtheoretical model (TTM) – a stage model for motivational and behaviour change.[10,11] Everyone screened received a colour print-out of their own profile including targets agreed for changing lifestyle. Information was offered on the Khush Dil activity programme where appropriate, and a copy of blood test results with a brief on the clinic intervention was sent to the GP. If deemed necessary, direct referral to the GP was made and minor medical queries were directed to a local clinician who offered project support on a consultation basis. Follow-up appointments to review progress and monitor health outcomes were planned on a 6–12 month time-scale.

Clinics run in partnership with voluntary organisations proved to be very effective and the support of South Asian workers was an important feature of their success. Voluntary organisation staff arranged the venue and structured clinic appointments thus ensuring good attendance with minimal default. Clinical screening and dietetic support were offered in tandem making effective use of project staff time. The informal setting provided a good platform for health promotion with clinic attendees often staying beyond their clinic appointments for social support and discussion. Discussions were geared towards cardiac health, often with a key focus on nutritional issues. Thus, an added value was brought to these interventions which promoted staff familiarity, knowledge and greater understanding of the client group. The sessions also highlighted the benefits of flexible working outside the medical centre setting.

In addition to in-house assessment, an independent Action Research project funded by the British Heart Foundation carried out a qualitative review of project activities over the first year. Feedback on the clinical service was very positive with time given to individual consultation highlighted as a particular benefit.[12]

Community lifestyle activities

A core programme of activities was organised and clinic attendees were channelled into these following clinic or dietetic assessment (Box 7.1). Individuals could also opt or be referred into another activity at any point during the project. Group courses offering a series of taster sessions in the different activities worked particularly well with established groups and with individuals who regularly attended groups run by voluntary agencies. Some participants were solely interested in screening or, in the case of local

Box 7.1 Activities offered via Khush Dil

- Introduction to cardiac risk factors & ELS training
- Introduction to diabetes
- Nutrition workshops
- Healthy cooking workshops
- Aerobic exercise for women
- Circuit training for men
- Paths to Health walking groups
- Jog Scotland walk/jog groups
- Stress management
- Smoking cessation
- Alcohol management
- Health promotion events including small group seminars, a fruit smoothie stall at the annual Edinburgh Asian Mela and two major Family Health Fairs run from local community venues

businesses, screening plus nutritional/dietetic input. A few people attended core exercise activities following information given at clinics, but the majority of participants in these were members of existing groups and this form of association emerged as a central factor governing confidence of participation and motivation to engage in lifestyle changes.

South Asian community workers were a key asset and sixteen people received training to support the development and running of the healthy lifestyle programme in the first year. Monitoring was implemented through numerical counts of activity sessions and attendance levels (Table 7.1). Questionnaires and group discussions were also employed to elicit participant feedback and self-assessment forms used for activity leaders to prompt reflective analysis of self-performance. Responses were affirmative with exercise-to-music classes for women and nutrition/cookery workshops particularly well received.

Table 7.1 Summary of lifestyle activities offered between September 2002 and July 2004

Activity	Total number of sessions + duration of session	Average number of participants per session	Total attendances
Walk programme	166 x 1hr	6	1022
Walk/jog programme	50 x 1hr	3	150
Women's exercise	149 x 1hr	7	1047
Men's exercise	23 x 1hr	4	94
Emergency life support	13 x 2hr	6/7	85
Nutrition workshops	31 x 2hrs	8	260
Stress management workshops	13 x 2hrs	6	78
CHD/diabetes workshops	5 x 2hr	10	48
Totals	450	Overall average per session = 6	2,784

Screening outcomes

To gauge the impact of Khush Dil activities, the health status of clinic attendees was recorded and compared over two time periods using a range of clinical health measurements and a lifestyle questionnaire. Health outcomes at each visit were compared to assess whether or not project interventions had a positive impact overall. Clinical data analysis has been carried out independently by staff at the University of Edinburgh and a joint paper reporting on outcomes is being prepared for publication in 2005. A brief summary of findings is presented here.

Cardiac risk factors

Standard parameters were used to identify CHD risk markers and clinic attendees (n=304) were rated in respect of individual risk factor occurrence. In the non-modifiable category, a strong prevalence of family history of diabetes and cardiovascular disease (c. 50% in each) was demonstrated. Several new cases of diabetes were diagnosed with the overall tally demonstrating one in five people with this condition. Further significant numbers returned raised random blood glucose levels.

In respect of non-modifiable factors, lack of exercise and overweight (87%) were the most frequently occurring. At initial consultation, 189 participants (62%) took part in no form of moderate exercise (30 minutes' duration or more) on a weekly basis and only 40 (13%) reported taking part in four or more moderate 30-minute sessions per week. Raised blood pressure, cholesterol levels and stress also presented as important areas for health improvement. Almost one in five people presented with a diagnosis of hypertension but a further quarter of the sample were found to have a systolic pressure of 140mmHg or higher and/or a diastolic pressure over 90mmHg.

At follow-up (n=140), individual risk factors were still very much in evidence but incidence had declined with statistically significant mean reductions recorded in respect of systolic and diastolic pressures, cholesterol levels, Body Mass Index (BMI), weight, salt and fat consumption, and activity levels. The number of people reporting to participate in moderate exercise more than four times a week had doubled whilst those taking less than one period of moderate exercise per week had reduced by almost half. These results demonstrate a significant shift in numbers engaging in moderate exercise with most participants making positive changes to increase their activity levels.

Collective risk scores

In addition to identifying individual risk factors, the CALM package[9] compiled a collective, user-friendly CHD risk rating (0–100) for each person who fell within one of three groupings:

- Low risk <20
- Moderate risk 20 – 50
- High risk >50

Table 7.2 shows that the mean collective modifiable risk score at first visit emerged as 28 (moderate risk). Using the CALM graphics as a visual guide, most clinic participants had agreed self-defined goals to improve their risk rating score out of 100, with the majority

Table 7.2 Mean risk ratings of participants using CALM thermometer scoring system

Collective modifiable risk score at:	Mean thermometer score rating:
1st attendance	28
Review	20
Target score	17

achieving these. The area with least success was weight reduction which is notoriously difficult to achieve. However, over 70% of people at least partially met their target and thus had achieved a degree of weight loss by the time of their review visit. The overall mean risk score dropped from 28 to 20 points, less than the overall mean target of 17 but demonstrating good progress towards this goal. Overall the numbers of participants falling within the high and moderate risk groupings had reduced at the review appointment (Fig.7.1). This is offset by an increase in numbers within the low risk rating category.

Motivational level/stage of change

A shift in motivational change between initial screening and follow-up was noted. Following the intervention, participants progressed from the early stages (pre-contemplation and preparation) of the model towards the later stages (action and maintenance). This seems to reflect the increased motivation of clinic attendees to make the healthy lifestyle changes agreed at the initial visit.

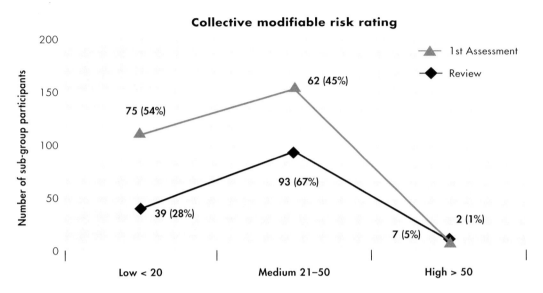

Fig. 7.1 Comparison of modifiable risk scores in sub-group at initial visit and review

Although sample numbers are not large (attendees: 1st assessment, n=304; follow-up, n=140), clinical findings show that most participants succeeded in making significant reductions to their CHD risk rating and did not set unrealistic goals in terms of health change. Clinical input, however, cannot be divorced from the range of health education and lifestyle activities that ran alongside, particularly in the areas of nutrition, exercise and general CHD/diabetes awareness. Thus, a number of strategies to support behaviour change were employed that repeatedly reinforced health messages in a variety of community settings. The challenge is now to find cost-effective and sustainable means of transferring the benefits of this project model into the wider mainstream.

Discussion

Government policy stresses the need to mainstream or standardise services, making these acceptable for all. The need to shape healthcare to improve equality of provision is in no doubt but guidance on how to achieve this in practical terms is less apparent. Mainstreaming is an ideological term that can be interpreted in a number of ways but at the heart of this concept lies a common recognition that the NHS needs to change the way existing services are delivered and new ones planned so that access for all people is improved.

In respect of CHD/Diabetes prevention for South Asians (and potentially, other high-risk BME groups), Khush Dil's experience recommends that services need to be partially targeted to effectively meet needs. This is necessary to develop appropriate cultural understandings, build positive relationships and increase confidence levels in people who are unfamiliar with UK health service structures and health promoting initiatives. Once groundwork has been laid, targeted services can then be gradually and systematically incorporated within general provisions via a process of reverse integration. This suggests that certain forms of service be developed around the specific needs of hard-to-reach communities but then, once a good confidence level has been attained, these services can be sensitively extended to include others.

Khush Dil has been an experimental project that sought to explore the meaning of culturally appropriate practice in respect of community-based CHD risk prevention for South Asians. Population numbers in Edinburgh are lower than in other major UK cities and work mainly revolved around numerous small groups, many of whom are affiliated to voluntary and religious organisations or local businesses. It emerged that working qualitatively with small pockets of people could, however, be very effective as momentum gathers over time with information spreading along community networks that are notably stronger in South Asian groupings than the population in general.

Our experience has highlighted many areas for health service improvement and major challenges to address in respect of CHD risk reduction. Modes of communication to meet the needs of people from different ethnic backgrounds present a real challenge. People preferred face-to-face contact and few were receptive to the written word. Many people had significant risk factors but little knowledge of ways to address these, and lack of compliance in taking medication was common because of poor understanding, despite regular contact with NHS services. Issues such as these have serious implications, not only for health information transfer and delivery but also for planning and administration of client contact. To organise clinic and lifestyle sessions, direct contact was most effective, using skilled bilingual workers to accurately convey messages, co-ordinate appointments and, very importantly, to motivate participation. The assurance of being with others who speak the same language and follow the same cultural norms is a key factor. Without a common language, effective information transfer is extremely difficult; thus, bilingual instructors with community development skills and the ability to promote cross-cultural communication are an obligatory requisite for mainstreaming.

Operating out of the traditional (GP/hospital) medical setting has given the advantage of de-medicalising care offered, and nurse-led clinics have focused on lifestyle change via the use of motivational interviewing and goal-setting techniques. One drawback of this mode of working, however, is that it is difficult to target or systematically prioritise an identified group on the basis of, for example, age, gender, or cardiac risk rating. This would, in theory, be better facilitated using a GP practice list, and is in accord with the National Service Framework for Coronary Heart Disease recommending that high-risk groups be targeted for priority screening interventions.[13]

Government policy currently places a strong emphasis on public health offering wider options for healthcare delivery than ever before. The medical perspective has often fallen short of recognising the bigger picture in the past but we now have a range of alternatives opening up that could strengthen and build upon existing health provisions to offer more wide-reaching and comprehensive modes of community-centred care. Voluntary organisations currently play a very important role in health care support for South Asian people, albeit via a somewhat fragmented and often indirect approach. With improved co-ordination of voluntary sector services working in conjunction with Public Health specialists, other community and social care workers, and dedicated medical support it should be possible to provide a systematic model of care that achieves health targets and is culturally sensitive to the needs of different groups.

Whichever path is chosen, effective mainstreaming will demand new forms of training and a focus on capacity building to develop the necessary workforce skills. Primary Care must develop greater cultural awareness amongst staff, to embrace support offered by specialist bodies, e.g. the National Resource Centre for Minority Ethnic Health in Scotland, and to work more closely with the BME voluntary sector. To achieve positive, long-lasting health impacts, regular, consistent contact is needed and this is unlikely to become a reality without focused effort in the short and medium terms. As the NHS possesses limited cultural competence at present, it is recommended that targeted community initiatives continue to be supported, to help reduce the high levels of diabetes and CHD that are so prevalent in South Asian populations.

Conclusion: key messages for CHD prevention work with South Asians

Khush Dil's experience dictates that an effective framework for CHD primary prevention needs to be strongly rooted in a community-outreach model of care backed by qualitative research to explore and monitor practical strategies for mainstreaming. Khush Dil messages for successful working in CHD prevention with South Asian people are outlined in Box 7.2.

A targeted community-based outreach approach to coronary risk prevention with South Asians, a high-risk population, can have beneficial health outcomes giving an impetus to develop similar primary and community care initiatives on a wider and more generalised basis. Working within the framework of Fair for All, the NHS is required to

---

Box 7.2 Key messages

- Mainstreaming & cultural competence are complex concepts demanding quality standards to guide their practical application
- Health initiatives of this kind need to be linked into larger CHD/Diabetes health frameworks to prevent isolation and ensure that learning is integrated within wider service provision
- Awareness of cultural variance and how this can influence patterns of working is vital to developing realistic levels of expectation in respect of outcomes
- Capacity building within the ME workforce is needed to increase skills and extend health messages across South Asian communities
- Fostering good relationships with local champions promotes vital links into community networks
- Outreach, community-based services run from familiar environments are a positive means of accessing people
- A varied health action programme connecting clinical and lifestyle sessions, seminars and events is the best way of achieving health successes
- Wider public health approaches need to run alongside the action programme to address more deep-rooted influences affecting health.

promote greater equity and mainstream current provisions. Mainstreaming, however, is an untested area and there is a need for specific research to monitor and evaluate the transfer of project learning and assess health-promoting strategies for clinical effectiveness and sustained behaviour change.

The reality of effective mainstreaming, from our experience of working with one (non-homogenous) high-risk grouping, will present major challenges. Quality frameworks that are grounded in a practical understanding of local, evidence-based experience are needed to support this process. We do not think it feasible that this can be realised without some level of targeted provision in the short and medium terms to bridge current inequalities and to facilitate a sensitive, phased progression into mainstream. This will need community outreach approaches that are culturally sensitive, flexible, and accessible (run from a familiar environment) and which crucially foster good relationships with the at-risk community. Perhaps most importantly the strategy will need to target multiple risk factors. Varied health action programmes connecting clinical and lifestyle sessions, seminars and events are the best way of achieving health success. Long-term success of such programmes will inevitably depend on an adequate resource base including a skilled and dedicated staff team supported by a strong commitment at senior management level.

Note: *A full account of Khush Dil work can be found in our project report on the Scottish Health on the Internet.*[14]

References

1. British Heart Foundation (2003). Coronary Heart Disease Statistics: South Asians and Heart Disease. *BHF* 2003.

2. Bhopal R, Unwin N, White M, Yallop J, Walker L, Alberti KGMM, Harland J, Patel S, Ahmad N, Turner C, Watson B, Kaur D, Kulkarnioer A, Laker M, Tavridou A. Heterogeneity of coronary heart disease risk factors in Indian, Pakistani, Bangladeshi, and European origin populations. *Br Med J* 1999; **319**: 215–220.

3. Kooner JS and Chambers JC. Conceptualising the causes of coronary heart disease in South Asians. In: Patel KCR and Bhopal RS (eds). *The Epidemic of Coronary Heart Disease in South Asian Populations: Causes and Consequences.* SAHF Publishers 2004.

4. Nazroo J Y and Karlsen S. Sociology of Health and Illness 2002; **24**(1): 1–20.

5. Carlisle-Pesic. The Heart of the Community. *Nursing Times* 2001; **97**(38): 26–7.

6. Scottish Executive (2001). Social Justice – A Scotland where Everyone Matters Annual Report 2001.

7. Scottish Executive Health Department (2001). Fair for All; Improving the Health of Ethnic Minority Groups and the Wider Community in Scotland.

8. Commission for Racial Equality in Scotland (2002). Code of Practice on the Duty to Promote Race Equality 2002.

9. CALM Corporation (2002). CALM Computer Assisted Lifestyle Management. CALMHeart V.4 Software Manual June 2002.

10. Prochaska JP and DiClemente CD. Stages and processes of self change of smoking: toward an integrative model of change. *Journal of Consulting and Clinical Psychology* 1983; **51**: 390–395.

11. Miller WR and Rollnick S. *Motivational Interviewing. Preparing people to change addictive behaviour.* New York & London. The Guildford Press 1991.

12. Bhatnagar A, Fischbacher C, McLaughlan L, and Netto G. Khush Dil Research Project: Final Report 2004.

13. Department of Health (2002). *Coronary Heart Disease: National Service Frameworks.* Chapter 1: Reducing heart disease in the population. London: HMSO.

14. http://www.nhslothian.scot.nhs.uk/publications/khushdil/summary.pdf

8
Mobilising the British Heart Foundation

Qaim Zaidi

Introduction

The British Heart Foundation's (BHF) interest in South Asian communities was stimulated by observations that South Asians living in the UK (Indians, Pakistanis, Bangladeshis and Sri Lankans) have premature mortality from coronary heart disease (CHD) and a higher overall rate compared with the UK white European population. Furthermore, this disparity in mortality rates between South Asians and white Europeans is increasing.[1] Finally, mainstream NHS campaigns were not being as effective in inducing lifestyle changes in South Asians as they were in the white European population.[2]

The aim of the BHF is to play a leading role in the fight against cardiovascular disease (CVD) so that it no longer remains a major cause of disability and premature death. The BHF has invested millions of pounds in research, care and support to achieve this aim. However, it has also been recognised that despite this commendable expenditure and effort, in order to make a significant difference within ethnic populations the BHF needs to target communities most affected by the pandemic of CHD, notably South Asians.

In 1999 the BHF organised a two-day workshop to consult health professionals, community health workers and community leaders from ethnic minorities to develop a strategy for the prevention and management of CHD in ethnic minority groups. The BHF then put into place an organisational structure that would allow it to draw upon expert opinion to guide its allocation of resources and to guide the development of culturally appropriate and multilingual resources. This involved the appointment of an ethnic strategy co-ordinator, charged with the responsibility for overseeing programmes, and a strategy committee comprised of experts who would help to direct the overall programme.

Following an active 5-year period in which a multitude of initiatives were supported by the BHF, a review in 2004 assessed progress that had been made and identified priorities for the future. The consensus was that work with South Asian groups would continue, but additional minority groups would also be targeted, e.g. Afro-Caribbean populations with a high prevalence of hypertension, and refugees and migrants from Eastern Europe.

In this paper, we look at some of the factors that specifically affect South Asian communities in terms of their relatively higher incidence of CHD, their relatively poor experience in managing it and also the issues present in accessing appropriate healthcare. We will highlight specific initiatives supported by the BHF in order to confront these issues and challenges. These initiatives have sought to educate both the patients and the wider target communities. The programmes developed have sought to reduce inequalities, encourage community involvement to engage in issues of real concern and remain cost effective.

This chapter focuses specifically on the British Heart Foundation activities to reduce the incidence of coronary heart disease, but the issues raised will also be relevant to other voluntary organisations such as the Stroke Association in relation to reducing the incidence, and raising awareness, of stroke.

Background

Factors contributing to the epidemic of CVD in South Asian populations have been discussed in earlier chapters. In addition to classical risk factors such as family history, diabetes, physical inactivity and smoking,[3] economic deprivation, stress, racism and diet are also important.[4]

A key aspect of programmes developed by the BHF is sensitivity to the heterogeneity of the South Asian population. The importance of this has been highlighted by Bhopal[4] who argues that the term South Asian is often used to refer to Indians, Pakistanis, Bangladeshis and Sri Lankans as one homogeneous group whereas, in reality, these populations show great diversity. Recognising the heterogeneity in South Asian populations is important when developing initiatives to combat CHD, e.g. smoking is less prevalent in Sikhs than in Hindus, whilst the reverse applies to alcohol consumption. This awareness is reflected in the tailored programmes highlighted later.

The BHF also appreciates that within South Asian communities there are differences in terms of education, employment, and awareness of CHD risk factors. Therefore we feel that our campaigns for the general population will also benefit South Asians. For example, the BHF annual 'Valentine's Day' and 'Heart Week' campaigns contain elements tailored to the South Asian population, as does the highly successful BHF 'Give Up Before You Clog Up' anti-smoking campaign, funded by the Department of Health.

Economic factors

As with the general population, an association between low social class and higher CVD mortality and risk factors has emerged in South Asians.[4,5] This socioeconomic gradient has direct implications for interventions undertaken by the BHF. The programmes supported focus on areas of economic deprivation, where needs in areas such as smoking cessation are greatest. Furthermore, the minority ethnic groups of people living in poor socioeconomic conditions are often those with communication and literacy issues, which serve as access barriers to healthcare. To address such issues we have developed the 'Health Advocates' programme, which is outlined in detail later in this paper.

Diet and physical activity

As discussed in earlier chapters, nutrition, physical inactivity and obesity are important risk factors in South Asians. Bangladeshi and Pakistani communities eat the least fruit and vegetables of all ethnic groups. Only 15% of Bangladeshi men and 16% of women consume fruit six or more times a week. Only 18% of Bangladeshi men and 7% of Bangladeshi women meet the current recommended physical activity levels. The BHF is aware of these factors and has targeted initiatives to address this.

Diabetes

Diabetes is a major risk factor for CHD and as discussed by Barnett and colleagues earlier in this text, South Asians living in the UK are five to six times more likely to develop type 2 diabetes. South Asians also develop diabetes on average ten years earlier than their white European counterparts.[6] Self-management of diabetes is poorer amongst South Asians and the risks associated with poor management of diabetes are not well understood by members of the community due to communication and cultural barriers.

Accessing health care

South Asians have been shown in several studies to have a lower awareness and knowledge of how to manage chronic conditions and CHD, compared to other ethnic groups.[7] The Health Survey of England indicates that CVD plays a significant part in health inequalities faced by black and minority ethnic groups (BMEG) and access to health information and advice is impaired by cultural and linguistic barriers.[8,9]

Feder et al[10] found that among patients deemed appropriate for angioplasty or coronary artery bypass grafting, South Asian patients were less likely to receive it than white European patients. These differences were independent of clinical need and were not wholly explained by variations in socioeconomic status or physician bias in recommending patients for revascularisation. Patient understanding and preference also play a role. In some areas, it is apparent that no attempt has been made to make communication accessible to ethnic minority patients, e.g. some diabetic clinics in areas with ethnic minority patients, where 40% had no adapted diet sheets and 34% had no hospital interpreter.[11] Despite obvious communication barriers there appears to be, at least in some regions, inadequate provision for ethnic minority needs.

Where an attempt has been made to cater for BMEG needs, this may not always take into account ethnic 'peculiarities'. Hawthorne[12] found that there are more complex communication problems, e.g. Pakistani Punjabi speakers preferring to read text in Urdu rather than in Punjabi since the former language is written in a script which they can understand whilst Punjabi is written in a script which is unfamiliar to Pakistani

Punjabis. According to Schott,[13] equitable access is not derived by offering the same service to all but by providing flexible services in which differing needs are identified and accommodated so that each individual benefits equally. As a result, the BHF is striving to develop services and resources according to the needs of various groups.

Initiatives supported by the BHF

We shall review some of the initiatives supported by the BHF, aiming to address the issues highlighted above. Appendix Tables A and B list some relevant recently funded BHF grant applications and we begin with a summary of resources that we have developed.

BHF resources

In 2000, the BHF undertook focus groups in London, Birmingham, Leicester and Bradford with various South Asian communities to ascertain:

- Target groups' knowledge of CHD risk factors, prevention and management
- Preferred format for resources
- Preferences in terms of language and design

Audiovisual aids

We found from these focus groups that there is clear preference for videos with real people (case studies) rather than written material. For that reason, we produced videos in Bengali, Punjabi, Gujarati, Urdu/Hindi and English for health professionals and carers. The videos which have been produced are:

- 'Living to prevent heart disease', which focuses on prevention and management of CHD.
- 'Get fit, keep fit and prevent heart disease', which focuses on physical activities one can do individually or in a group. The video shows how physical activity can be fun and help to improve fitness, reduce stress and prevent CHD.

- 'Heart Surgery', which seeks to inform and reassure patients and their families about cardiac surgery. Case histories show patients who have had cardiac surgery and their recovery after the surgery.

- 'Cardiac Rehabilitation', which explains cardiac rehabilitation and its importance in recovery. It shows the speedy recovery of patients who had joined a structured rehabilitation programme.

- A video on sex and heart disease. After a heart attack or cardiac surgery, many patients and their partners are anxious about resuming a sexual relationship. This video addresses these anxieties and explains how and where to get help. It reassures patients and their partners that resuming a sexual relationship is part of their recovery.

Booklets

We have also developed two booklets in Urdu, Hindi, Gujarati, Bengali, Punjabi and English:

- 'Looking After your Heart', which deals with the prevention and management of CHD, and

- 'Medicines for Heart', which explains drug regimes, the reasons for taking certain medication and drug side-effects.

Other initiatives related to the development of resources were as follows:

- We have awarded two grants to the Chinese Healthy Living Centre, one to develop a training programme for Chinese takeaway chefs on how to make healthier food, and the other to develop a training video.

- A grant was made to Camden PCT to develop a video on CHD prevention for the Bangladeshi community.

- In 2001 we worked with an Asian television channel to produce a series of programmes on CHD prevention and management.

Media utilisation

We have made extensive use of Asian media. All of our campaigns have been widely publicised on Asian television and radio channels.

Health advocates

In broad terms, this project deals with CHD prevention and management for minority ethnic communities. Communication in the English language is a significant issue. In one population, Wilson et al[14] found that only 26% spoke English and that only 20% could read English. CHD patients using interpreter services may have a limited comprehension about CHD. Terms translated into their mother tongue may have little or no meaning unless these terms are explained. This project deals with the importance of training bilingual link workers and advocacy workers who work with minority ethnic communities as interpreters. These workers interface with health professionals such as cardiologists, General Practitioners, nurses and cardiac rehabilitation nurses.

Advocacy is based on the recognition that there is an unequal relationship between patients and health service staff. For certain groups of patients, it is difficult to negotiate what happens to them in hospital on their own terms. The role of the advocacy worker is to find out from staff the answers to the patients' questions and to explain to the patient the options that are available.

Health advocates are not simply interpreters. They can inform people about health services, help patients and their families make informed decisions about their care, and work with health professionals to develop culturally appropriate services. They are essential partners in improving the health of the most deprived communities. The King's Fund mapping exercise states that 80% of health advocacy is provided by voluntary organisations; this makes it more important for the BHF to train advocates in the prevention and management of CHD.

Using Melas to target Asian communities

Melas (or South Asian fairs) are now among the most popular cultural events in the British summer. Like 'Chicken Tikka Masala' they have become an integral part of summer festivals in many British towns and cities. Melas have their origins on the Indian subcontinent, where they mark key events in the local agricultural and religious calendar. Today, many British local authorities and town councils have adopted these Melas as part of their local community development, communication and diversity strategies. In 2003, over 850,000 (37% of the total 2.5 million UK South Asian population) had attended at least one such fair. The 2001 Census also shows that the BMEG population in the UK is geographically concentrated in certain areas and Melas held in these areas are likely to reach significant numbers of these communities.

Health promotion undertaken at Melas needs to focus on areas where the epidemiological evidence points to an important need in the South Asian population. In the Mela project, we have provided information, advice, counselling, screening and support in a culturally and linguistically sensitive manner to the various groups via qualified and well-trained multilingual health advisers, e.g. pharmacists, nurses, smoking cessation advisers, dieticians, and experts in physical activity and counsellors who are supported by self-help material and resources in over nine languages. We have also worked with various Primary Care Trusts (PCTs) and Diabetes UK to raise awareness of diabetes and its management. With such partnerships, we have provided BMEG with resources such as videos and leaflets in various languages, covering topics such as healthy eating, increasing physical activity, reducing weight and managing CHD and diabetes, in addition to quitting smoking. The Melas have also provided us with an opportunity to offer a 'Health MOT' using testing kits to measure cholesterol, blood pressure and blood glucose levels, and CO monitors to assess smoking status.

Reaching women and the young from ethnic minorities is a challenge for health professionals. An important benefit of using Melas as a portal for communication and access into South Asian communities is that they provide an excellent opportunity to reach these groups without interrupting their daily schedule and where they have time to talk to health professionals. In the case of the young, Melas can also reach all ranges of the age spectrum. For example, the BHF recruits members for the Artie Beat Club at Melas. This is a BHF initiative for 7–11-year-old children where club members receive an Artie Beat magazine every four months which contains important information on, amongst other things, diet and exercise.

The pharmacists at our stands have encouraged people to make use of local pharmacies, which can play a major role in the prevention and management of CHD. Their role has been acknowledged by the National Service Framework on CHD.[15] In many inner city areas, pharmacists are from a South Asian background and speak several Asian languages, an asset which can play a major role in prevention and better management of CHD and diabetes.

In our work during the Mela and Ramadan projects, we came to know of many CHD patients who were not aware of the importance of or reasons for taking certain medicines. For example, many South Asians assume that aspirin is solely for headaches and we heard of several patients who had stopped taking aspirin because they did not have any headache! We also heard of instances where patients had stopped taking medication or reduced their dosages during Ramadan without consulting their physician. We hope that our 'Medicines for Heart' leaflet will provide such patients with the necessary information to manage their drugs with confidence.

Places of worship project

The BHF works with Asian Quitline and various places of worship to promote a healthy lifestyle, raise awareness of CHD prevention and management, and provide training in cardiopulmonary resuscitation (CPR). In certain South Asian communities, places of worship provide an ideal opportunity to promote health and to engage with hard-to-reach groups. We have found the following distinct advantages:

• For many first generation immigrants, places of worship provide the only opportunity to meet and socialise. In some communities, these places provide health promoters with opportunities to engage families and their social networks.

- Messages may become more credible if delivered in a sacred place and sometimes even more effective if they are delivered by a priest trained in basic health promotion. These religious scholars are able to relate our message to the teaching of their religion, thus making the message even more effective.

- These events are cost effective as one large place of worship may hold up to six thousand people.

- Working with places of worship offers the BHF an opportunity to work in partnership with the local community, PCT and related organisations.

In this programme, we also fund and participate in a proactive Ramadan campaign where we have been training Imams (mosque prayer leaders) in basic lifestyle issues such as diet, smoking and exercise. We have offered this training in London, Manchester, Birmingham, Walsall and Bradford. In the holy month of Ramadan, Muslims who are fasting do not eat, drink, smoke or have sex from dawn to dusk. As it is a festive period, food high in fat and sugar content is widely available, emphasising the need for dietary advice. The month also provides an ideal opportunity for Muslims to stop smoking. By training Imams, key people who have subsequently disseminated our healthy lifestyle messages, we have reached thousands of Muslims, a community which is considered the most disadvantaged in terms of economic well being and health.

Summary

In summary, we have seen that there is a range of factors that could possibly explain the relatively high levels of CVD amongst South Asians and that there are a range of initiatives that can raise community awareness of these issues. However, as identified in this paper, success in one area with one community cannot be assumed to be a recipe for success elsewhere. Individual programmes need to be tailored to account for the needs of each target group in order to be effective.

References

1. www.heartstats.org

2. British Heart Foundation coronary heart disease statistics (2004).

3. Zaidi QM. Smoking and smoking cessation in South Asian communities. In: Patel KCR and Bhopal RS (eds). *The Epidemic of Coronary Heart Disease in South Asian Populations: Causes and Consequences*. SAHF Publishers 2004.

4. Bhopal RS. Coronary heart disease in South Asians: the scale of the problem and the challenge. In: Patel KCR and Bhopal RS (eds). *The Epidemic of Coronary Heart Disease in South Asian Populations: Causes and Consequences*. SAHF Publishers 2004.

5. Department of Health press release: 'Secretary of State launches battle-plan for war on heart disease'. Published: 6/3/2000. Reference no: 2000/0130.

6. Nicholl CG, Levy JC, Mohan V, Rao PV, Mather HM. Asian diabetes in Britain: a clinical profile. *Diabet Med* 1986; **3**: 257–260.

7. Griffiths C, Kaur G, Gantley M, Feder G, Hillier S, Goddard J, Packe G. Influences on hospital admission for asthma in South Asian and white adults: qualitative interview study. *Br Med J* 2001; **323**: 962.

8. Department of Health. Health Survey of England, Minority Ethnic Groups. 1999.

9. Health Education Authority. The Second Black and Minority Ethnic Groups (BMEG) Lifestyle Survey. 2000.

10. Feder G, Crook AM, McGee P, Banerjee S, Timmis AD, Hemingway H. Ethnic differences in invasive management of coronary disease: prospective cohort study of patients undergoing angiography. *Br Med J* 2002; **324**: 511–516.

11. Mello M. Plugging the gap. *Nursing Times* 1992; **88** (43): 34–6.

12. Hawthorne K. Asian diabetics attending a British hospital clinic – a pilot study to evaluate their care. *British Journal of General Practice* 1990; **40**: 243–247.

13. Schott A. Culture, Religion and Childbearing in a Multiracial society. In: *A handbook for health professionals*. Butterworth Heinemann 2004.

14. Wilson E, Wardle EV, Chandel P, Walford S. Diabetes education: an Asian perspective. *Diabetic Medicine* 1993; **19**: 177–180.

15. National Service Framework for Coronary Heart Disease 2000.

Appendix Table A   Recently funded BHF initiatives relevant to South Asian CHD

Project title and research organisation	Summary of aims
Primary prevention of CHD in South Asian children in secondary schools University of Leicester in partnership with 6 inner city schools where pupils are predominantly of South Asian origin	To improve healthy lifestyle habits of the study population by determining levels of healthy eating and physical activity in secondary school children of South Asian ethnic origin and their families and to develop and evaluate a programme to improve these levels.
The Heartnet project The Open University, Whipps Cross University Trust and Quit	Based on the proposition that social factors are an important element in cardiac rehabilitation and, furthermore, that health professionals in making use of social networks need to pay attention to the way in which interpersonal communications are used in order to maximise their effectiveness. The project will involve working with cardiac rehabilitation patients and influence their social networks as a means of helping patients better manage their condition – thus helping with secondary prevention. This approach allows health professionals to disseminate information to a wider community which, because of the social and familial ties with the patient, is also likely to be at risk of CHD, thereby aiding primary prevention.
Dil ke Baat Staffordshire University and Palffrey Community Association, Walsall, Walsall Health Authority	To develop an Expert Patient Programme for South Asians with CHD. The programmes will include secondary prevention of CHD in primary care and cardiac rehabilitation. The project will help redesign existing services rather than seek to address the complex problems of inadequate services.
Ealing Coronary Risk Prevention Programme Ealing Hospital NHS Trust; Gurdwara Siri Guru Singh Sabha, Southall; Vishwa Hindu Temple, Southall; and Central Jamia Mosque, Southall	To investigate if National Service Framework (NSF) targets for CHD prevention can be improved among South Asians in Southall, through: 1 systematic identification of CHD patients, structured assessment of their risk factors, patients' possession of results, and therapeutic recommendations to patients' GPs based on NSF targets 2 additional specialist led CHD Nurse intervention in Primary Care

Appendix Table A (continued) Recently funded BHF initiatives relevant to South Asian CHD	
Project title and research organisation	**Summary of aims**
Coronary Artery Disease in South Asians Prevention (CADISAP) Dr S Gupta, Whipps Cross University Hospital	Cardiac rehabilitation (CR) can make a substantial difference, reducing mortality by 20%–30%. Despite these benefits, uptake of CR is especially low in ethnic minority groups. NSF for CHD 2000 states that services should be accessible and acceptable to all users. Uptake of services which are culturally appropriate is higher. The BHF is keen to increase uptake of CR services by minority ethnic groups. We have funded several CR programmes for South Asian groups. The CADISAP study is partly funded by the BHF. It is a unique study which set out to examine the impact of culturally specific interventions on the uptake and adherence to CR programmes. It is a multidisciplinary programme which includes education, psychological support, dietary advice, supervised exercise training and smoking cessation support given over a 12-week period. The study has demonstrated that culturally appropriate CR programmes can significantly improve uptake and adherence.
Fair and equal access to cardiac rehabilitation in Leicester	This project offers fair and equal access to cardiac rehabilitation services for South Asian patients, achieved by recruiting and training link workers from these communities in basic prevention and management of CHD and to enhance phase 1 and 2 of rehabilitation for South Asian communities.
Planning and delivering equitable cardiac rehabilitation in Newham	The rehabilitation team identified communication barriers as the most important cause of lower uptake of cardiac rehabilitation. Therefore they worked closely with the well-established advocacy service to produce a video, audio tapes and leaflets in eight languages covering various topics relating to healthy lifestyle and management of CHD. The project has been very successful in delivering the service to ethnic minorities.

Appendix Table B   Recent academic grant applications funded by the BHF relating to ethnicity and cardiovascular disease

Applicant and Institution	Details of Project
Professor Nish Chaturvedi University College London	Ethnic differences in macrovascular and microvascular function and their relation to hypertensive target organ damage
Professor Nish Chaturvedi St Mary's Hospital, London	Ethnic differences in macrovascular and microvascular structure and function associated with diabetes
Professor Nish Chaturvedi University College London	Differences between South Asians and Europeans in risk, distribution and determinants of atherosclerosis in the coronary and peripheral vessels
Professor Nish Chaturvedi St Mary's Hospital, London	Cardiovascular morbidity and mortality in an ethnically diverse cohort
Dr Yanbin Dong St George's Hospital Medical	Investigation of genetic determinants of sodium channel activity as a cause of high blood pressure in African-Caribbean people
Professor Alun Hughes St Mary's Hospital, London	Endothelial progenitor cells as a mediator of ethnic differences in cardiovascular risk in South Asians and Europeans
Dr Mark Kearney & Professor Ajay Shah King's College London	Exploring the mechanisms underlying endothelial dysfunction in Asian men
Dr John Oldroyd University of Manchester	Do maternal glycaemic status, diet and growth from birth to 2 years influence coronary risk factors in Pakistani and European infants?
Professor J Scott Imperial College London	Human genetic variation underlying risk of insulin resistance and type 2 diabetes in Indian Asian and Northern European men
Total of nine applications selected	**Total award** £2,390,595

9
Mobilising the Department of Health

Kiran CR Patel and Roger Boyle

Introduction

The National Health Service (NHS) was founded on the principle of equal access for the entire population it serves. With the advent of globalisation and migration, society has become truly diverse and this presents a significant challenge to the NHS and its workforce. Access and inequity issues remain at the forefront of our minds when it comes to discussing the needs of ethnic groups. Health needs assessments must therefore form the backbone of service delivery to ethnic populations. Interaction with all communities is essential to optimise healthcare delivery, and sharing of experiences is also invaluable. The NHS prides itself on striving to deliver equality, diversity and respect to the population it serves.

Coronary heart disease (CHD) is just one of the many diseases where there exists a difference in prevalence and incidence of disease between South Asians and the general population. Mortality rates from CHD are approximately 50% higher in South Asians than in the general population.[1] In addition, the difference in death rates between South Asian populations and the general population is increasing because mortality rates in South Asians are not falling as fast. Similar disparities are also in evidence for stroke.

The National Service Framework for coronary heart disease

Nearly 5 years after publication of the National Service Framework (NSF) for CHD,[2] heart disease remains a high priority for the NHS. The target to reduce death rate from CHD by 40% by 2010 is realistic and is likely to be achieved. The use of disease registers is beginning to ensure that those at high risk of developing heart disease receive appropriate advice regarding prevention strategies. The use of statin therapy has increased exponentially, with over 2 million people in the UK now in receipt of these drugs, and access to the drugs has also increased with the advent of over-the-counter availability of statins. As a consequence, several thousand lives per year are being saved.

Many areas of the NSF have provided improved services for all patients, e.g.

- Better and faster treatment of myocardial infarction and angina
- Faster diagnosis of angina in Rapid Access Chest Pain Clinics
- Reduced waiting times for angioplasty and cardiac surgery
- Improved cardiac rehabilitation
- Improved prevention strategies and identification of 'at risk' individuals.

Stroke services

Standard Five of the Older People's NSF published in 2001 outlined a programme of action for the NHS to reduce the incidence of stroke in the population and to ensure that those who have had a stroke have prompt access to integrated care services. The NSF has helped kick-start the widespread development of specialist stroke services. Where specialist stroke services were a rarity ten years ago, they are now in place everywhere. More patients are now seen by stroke specialist services than ever before.

A National Audit Office report published on 16th November 2005 showed that notable progress has been made from a low starting point and recommended further improvements in preventing stroke and treating and managing stroke patients, in line with recent evidence. In response the Department of Health has announced that work will begin on a new stroke strategy which will deliver the newest treatments and improve the care that stroke patients receive. Early action will include spreading examples of best practice and building a future generation of clinical champions through a programme to expand stroke physician training numbers.

Smoking cessation services

Smoking cessation services continue to provide invaluable advice to all groups and the NHS Smoking Helpline and the British Heart Foundation (BHF) funded Asian Quitline have provided an invaluable service to South Asian populations to date. In addition, a comprehensive tobacco control strategy is supported by government, e.g. media campaigns, legislation to ban tobacco advertising, promotion and sponsorship, larger warnings on cigarette packets and the removal of misleading terms such as 'low tar' or 'lights'.

Dietary advice

Initiatives to improve diet are well under way. Policies to improve school meals (given added impetus by Jamie Oliver in the recent past) are in development, with the aim that these should provide a third of the weekly fibre and protein for schoolchildren and also be low in sugar and salt content. The School Fruit and Vegetable Scheme and Food in Schools programmes have promoted healthy eating to schoolchildren. The impact of such initiatives on CHD, stroke and cancer will become apparent in the years to come.

Physical activity

Initiatives to increase physical activity are in abundance. With the increasing recognition of the importance of multi-agency working, a multi-faceted approach to tackling inactivity and its major consequence, obesity, is under way. There are now in excess of 700 GP exercise referral schemes prescribing physical activity to improve health. Pilot projects such as LEAP (Local Exercise Action Pilots) and Walking the Way to Health have been in existence for over a year now.

Tackling inequalities

There are several initiatives specifically addressing health inequalities and these have a particular focus on minority ethnic groups. Sustainable improvements in health and services for ethnic minority populations are key to the success of these initiatives. The NHS Plan[3] published in 2000 sets out ambitious plans to transform the quality of services, tackle health inequalities and deliver patient-centred, easily accessible services for all. The PCT-led Race for Health[4] aims to implement models of excellence and partnership, working with ethnic minority communities in implementing the Race Relations (Amendment) Act 2000.[5] Standards for Better Health[6] describes the standards that all healthcare organisations will be expected to meet in terms of safety, clinical and cost-effectiveness, governance, patient focus, accessibility and responsive care. These standards ensure that all parts of the target population are served and therefore inequalities must be addressed. The NHS Improvement Plan[7] includes a focus on public health, reducing inequalities and promoting cooperation between organisations to tailor best care for individual patients. Choosing Health,[8] a Public Health White Paper, aims to ensure that people have access to information and opportunities to eat more healthily, exercise more and smoke less. Already, the drive to smoke-free public places has taken on significant impetus.

Barriers to access

Many barriers are not unique to South Asians and must be addressed whenever inequalities are being challenged, e.g.:

- Poor health
- Lack of time
- Absent support network
- Transport issues
- Interpreting service requirements and longer consultations
- Culturally appropriate service provision, e.g. single-sex exercise classes
- Suitable health promotion materials.

There are several tools available for planning, delivering and assessing services, e.g. Health Equity Audits (which must take into account the different needs and inequalities within the local population served by PCTs),[9] and Healthcare Needs Assessments (valuable for those involved in commissioning services),[10] which ask the following questions:

- With what population or patients are we concerned?
- What services are currently provided?
- What is the evidence for effectiveness and cost-effectiveness of these services?
- What is the optimum configuration of these services?

Summary

The NHS must clearly work in partnership with communities and voluntary sector organisations to achieve the standards of service South Asian and other ethnic minority populations expect. The Khush Dil project described in an earlier chapter by Mathews is one of many projects around the UK aimed at addressing inequalities. Many of these projects are highlighted in a Department of Health publication[11] launched in December 2004 at the SAHF conference which forms the basis for this article. Not only do these projects tackle ethnicity but socioeconomic deprivation too, often at the heart of inequalities. The CHD NSF itself requires all NHS organisations to ensure that the services they provide are acceptable and accessible to the people they serve, regardless of ethnicity. Cultural, religious and linguistic sensitivity is at the heart of addressing acceptability and accessibility. Where barriers are identified, these must be tackled.

A great deal of work is already under way to improve access to services for South Asian communities, but clearly, more also needs to be done in terms of research, education and service development and delivery. The NHS is committed to playing an integral part in ameliorating health inequalities and despite the significant efforts to date, believes more can and will be done to achieve the objectives discussed in this chapter.

References

1. Coronary heart disease statistics 2004: British Heart Foundation Statistics www.heartstats.org

2. National Service Framework for Coronary Heart Disease www.dh.gov.uk/publications

3. NHS Plan www.dh.gov.uk

4. Race for Health www.dh.gov.uk

5. Race Relations (Amendment) Act 2000 www.dh.gov.uk

6. Standards for Better Health www.dh.gov.uk

7. NHS Improvement Plan www.dh.gov.uk

8. Choosing Health, a Public Health White Paper www.dh.gov.uk

9. Health Equity Audit www.dh.gov.uk/PolicyandGuidance

10. Health Care Needs Assessment http://hcna.radcliffe-oxford.com

11. Heart Disease and South Asians: Delivering the National Service Framework for Coronary Heart Disease www.dh.gov.uk

10
Overview of South Asian coronary heart disease and the road ahead:
an overview of the SAHF 2004 Conference

Raj S Bhopal

Introduction

In the 30 years since Tunstall-Pedoe and colleagues[1] first demonstrated a high incidence of heart attack in 'Asians' (presumably mainly Bangladeshis) in East London, UK research and practice has made vast progress. The finding corroborated work from overseas, most notably the study by Adelstein and colleagues[2] showing mortality in South African Indians (presumably a mix of South Asians) that was substantially higher than in whites. From my potentially biased view the UK has taken the global lead. There is, I believe, more known about the causes and consequences of the surprisingly high risk of coronary heart disease (CHD) in South Asians in the UK than anywhere else in the world. The research base may even exceed that in India. Yet, as this book shows, and as clinicians and observers of South Asian communities know, neither the mystery of causation, nor the challenge of control, has been solved.

The central mystery is this one: South Asians living in traditional rural ways on the Indian subcontinent have not been characterised as particularly susceptible to CHD (or even diabetes). Yet, on migration to urban centres worldwide these diseases are epidemic e.g. in the UK, South Asians' mortality from CHD exceeds even the incredibly high rates afflicting the local population – itself notorious for its susceptibility to this disease. Usually, migrant populations' rates of disease converge towards those of the population as a whole. Overshooting the mark, as here, is unusual. This overshooting is also seen in South Asians with diabetes, and stroke – for the latter it is less surprising because, unlike CHD, stroke is strongly associated with poverty.

Most medical mysteries that relate to chronic diseases with a long natural history (the period between exposure to causes and the outcomes and their consequences) are complex. Early hypotheses that focused on insulin resistance and diabetes – pioneered by Cruickshank[3] and McKeigue,[4] separately – have stood the test of time, but they paint an incomplete picture, even leaving aside the equally compelling mystery of why there should be such an excess of these problems and how they might cause CHD. The picture is complex, but at its core is the unbelievably rapid change to a lifestyle characterised by ample nutrition that leads to a huge rise in cholesterol, blood pressure and weight gain (particularly around the waist).[5] This is accompanied by a sedentary lifestyle, and in men if not women, a level of tobacco consumption that needs tackling – especially in Muslim men.[6] Even this is only part of the picture. The low birth weight of South Asian babies, the high levels of homocysteine that probably reflect B12 deficiency, the high level of exposure to infections, the use of specific substances in food, the stresses and strains of migration and occupational change, and, of course, genes are some of the additional factors in the equation.[7] We look forward to a future SAHF conference where the summary ends with a simple one-sentence account of the high rates of CHD in South Asians. Our present conference has taken us one step in this lengthy journey.

The conference: a personal account

This was the second SAHF conference on the topic of CHD – an indicator of the high priority that is rightly attached to this problem. What were some of the differences from the first one, and what new challenges did it throw up?

The conference opened up with a proclamation by the Chairman (Shah) that our first goal is to serve our community and patients and that research must be subservient to this goal. That our goal is embraced by the UK's health care and research institutions was emphasised by the words, deeds and presence of the Chairman of NICE (Rawlins), the National Clinical Director (Tsar) for Heart Disease (Boyle), the Board Programme Manager of the MRC (Sarna) and the Medical Director of the BHF (Weissberg). Subsequent to the conference the SAHF has become involved in six NICE groups. Boyle reminded us that CHD mortality, if not morbidity, is tumbling and that within decades CHD in some countries could be a disease of the past. He focused us on the challenging target of reducing inequalities (by 40%). With this in mind, and the Department of Health's structures for tackling race inequality, it does appear that SAHF and the Department of Health share a common goal on this front.

Sarna made no empty promises, rather he reminded us that research funding is highly competitive, and that scientific issues drive the funding though strategy plays a part. This accurate analysis merits widespread reflection. Sarna challenged us to pinpoint the important questions. Indeed, we must do so. The problem is that one usually needs to establish a foundation for research. For example, there are numerous cohort studies in the world, but virtually none that examine risk factor–outcome relations in South Asians. In their analysis of 71 cardiovascular studies in North America and Europe, Ranganathan and Bhopal found none had any data for South Asians.[8] The full paper describing the study will be published shortly in the journal *Public Library of Science*. Establishing such a cohort study has been a formidable challenge – attempts have failed to win funding – and we are very fortunate that such a study, called LOLIPOP, is under way. Kooner told the conference about incredible work that is in the field in Southall. The target is 24,000 people screened for an array of risk factors and followed up for cardiovascular outcomes. The sample will be 50:50 South Asians and Europeans. Smaller numbers are being intensively phenotyped. This study, which is well on the way towards its target, deserves to be better known. Kooner told me that the name LOLIPOP (in idiomatic English lollipop means a very small amount of resource) was chosen to reflect the sparse resources he had to conduct the study and only later did the words for the acronym come to mind. We need to reflect on why a problem that was identified in 1975 in the UK[1] was not immediately addressed using the powerful cohort design, and why, eventually, a study was started without funding from the research councils and major charities. There are serious questions about the laissez-faire competitive model of researcher-led funding system. It is dependent on champions for a cause. South Asians are lucky that champions have emerged. Where are the studies for other ethnic minority groups in the UK?

The absence of cohort data is problematic, not only for causal understanding but also for practice. Clinical practice is now founded on risk prediction models. If risk of CHD mortality or serious morbidity such as heart attack exceeds the pragmatically chosen threshold of 30% over 10 years the patient is to be managed with statins, among other therapies. I presented an analysis of the predictive accuracy of the Framingham, FINRISK and SCORE models and showed that these were wanting. Cohort data are sorely needed to produce more valid models. As this work showed, reduction of risk factors does promise a great deal in South Asians.[9] These models performed even worse in predicting stroke.

Consultant neurologist, Sharma, reviewed stroke in South Asians but uncovered comparatively little information, so he and colleagues did a small but important study on stroke in East London. The message was stark – there is a great deal of room for improvement for all ethnic groups. With stroke rates in South Asians that are in even greater excess than CHD we can foresee the need for a series of SAHF conferences to move this field on.[10]

How to move from debate to action was among the many questions posed by the Chairman of the BHF Ethnic Health Strategy Committee (Gupta). Among the mind-blowing facts that he presented was one not easily forgotten: a single samosa – that staple of South Asian hospitality – contains 26 grams of fat. Even if the one he referred to was an atherosclerotic monster and an aberration, this is still worrying. There are so many such delicacies that were rare, precious and occasional in the Indian subcontinent context, which have now become everyday fare, as cost in relation to income has tumbled. How are we to move from the current culture, where delicious samosas are central to the hospitality that cements relationships, to their replacement with, say, pears and apples? That is a formidable health behaviour challenge.

The research director of the Health Development Agency (Kelly) was able to enlighten us that health behaviour change models do work, and that no one model was demonstrably superior to another. So, the SAHF and its allies can choose from the health belief model, the stages of change model or the theory of planned behaviour model. Unfortunately, most of the research underpinning the models is from N. America, and none is on South Asians. Kelly reminded us that key to behaviour change is an understanding of the life-worlds of the population that we are hoping to help. In this challenge we see a huge role for SAHF – it is bringing together experts on the life-worlds of South Asians and subject matter experts – an alliance that is indispensable.

The Heartlands Hospital in Birmingham serves a very large South Asian population and is well served to undertake intervention-based research as described by Barnett. The UK Asian Diabetes Study is in his words the MRFIT for South Asians. It is a trial of protocol-driven behaviour and therapeutic management of South Asians with diabetes. The pilot study has shown that change is possible and the definitive one will assess costs and effectiveness. The findings are likely to influence practice very greatly.

Four practitioners offered insight from their community- and general-practice-based services. From Wolverhampton (Sahmi) came a story illustrating the immense difficulties in bringing about change in the face of denial, resistance, illiteracy and lack of cultural knowledge among so many practitioners. The pioneering Project Dil (Farooqi) has been going since 1999 and is now an integral part of the NHS-funded services in Leicester. Its core strategy was peer education, led by 45 students funded by the project to take the message to the people. Building on the Project Dil idea, the Edinburgh Khush Dil Project (Mathews) has combined clinic screening and community education elements. Evaluation has shown that it is effective in reducing cardiovascular risk. The challenge of embedding the learning from the project into routine NHS service is greater than predicted and solutions are currently being tested. Complementing these local projects is the work of the BHF Ethnic Health Strategy Committee and its key Ethnic Strategy Officer (Zaidi). A steady stream of educational materials and other initiatives is being disseminated, both directly to the public and to practitioners. Perhaps the most heartening development is the relative ease with which the BHF has accepted the need to integrate the ethnic health dimension into its work.

Future directions

The first conference in 2001 emphasised the scientific issues, the epidemiological perspectives and the public health consequences. The second conference in 2004 emphasised the practical experiences of implementing research, using the data, and changing professional practice and individuals' behaviours. The third conference in December 2005 will spur the development of more effective guidelines.

The work to date sends us in three major directions. The first and foremost is to use the knowledge we have to stem the loss of lives, livelihood and health from this preventable epidemic. It is quite probable that by applying what we already know we could reduce CHD by 80% in the South Asian community. This only needs focused policies, plans, resources and actions that mobilise communities and health professionals to a common cause. Of course, this is easy to write but hard to achieve.

The second direction is to learn more. This requires large-scale, collaborative and innovative research. Work is needed on a broad front with a balance between basic science and applied research. The gaps need to be filled, even if such work is not cutting edge in the sense that it has been done in white populations before. The challenge is too big for researchers alone. We need help from our communities, from leaders and from statutory and voluntary funders. Statutory research funders and the NHS, in partnership with the political, religious and social leaders of our communities, need to call for such work and give it due priority. South Asian communities need to participate eagerly – that means we need to make them more aware of why research is important and make it easy for them to play a part. Leaders of South Asian communities have a huge and urgent role to play. There is a great deal of wealth in the South Asian community. Some of this would be well spent in acts of much-needed philanthropy. These are too rare in the field of medical research, though one cannot deny the generosity to other causes (particularly religious). Both researchers and practitioners require such philanthropy – it has been, and continues to be, an integral part of research funding in Britain for hundreds of years.

Third, we need to generalise our learning. South Asians are part of a world community. Research and practice in UK South Asians have lessons for the UK as a whole, and particularly for other ethnic minority groups. Our work also has implications for South Asians worldwide, including the Indian subcontinent. SAHF has international objectives. As a small and new organisation the SAHF must not, however, be overambitious. The saying goes that you must not run before you learn to walk. SAHF is a toddler that is walking steadily. Perhaps it is time to reach out, holding hands with international organisations with like goals, so that it can take the giant strides it wants and needs to more swiftly.

References

1. Tunstall-Pedoe H, Clayton D, Morris JN, Bridge W, McDonald L. Coronary heart-attack in East London. *Lancet* 1975; **2**: 833–8.

2. Adelstein AM. Some aspects of cardiovascular mortality in South Africa. *Brit J Prev Soc Med* 1963; **17**: 29–40.

3. Cruickshank JK, Cooper J, Burnett M, MacDuff J, Drubra U. Ethnic differences in fasting plasma C-peptide and insulin in relation to glucose tolerance and blood pressure. *Lancet* 1991; **338**: 842–7.

4. McKeigue PM, Shah B, Marmot MG. Relation of central obesity and insulin resistance with high diabetes prevalence and cardiovascular risk in South Asians. *Lancet* 1991; **337**: 382–6.

5. Bhatnagar D, Anand IS, Durrington PN, Patel DJ, Wander GS, Mackness MI et al. Coronary risk factors in people from the Indian subcontinent living in west London and their siblings in India. *Lancet* 1995; **345**: 405–9.

6. Bhopal R, Vettini A, Hunt S, Wiebe S, Hanna L, Amos A. Review of Prevalence data in, and evaluation of methods for cross cultural adaptation of, UK surveys on tobacco and alcohol in ethnic minority groups. *Br Med J* 2004; **328**: 76–80.

7. Bhopal R. Coronary heart disease in South Asians: The scale of the problem and the challenge. In: Patel KCR and Bhopal R (eds). *The epidemic of cononary heart disease in South Asian populations: causes and consequences.* First ed. Birmingham: SAHF Publishers 2004; 1–18.

8. Ranganathan M, Bhopal R. Exclusion and inclusion of non-white racial and ethnic minority groups in 65 key North American and European cardiovascular cohort studies. *Ethnicity & Health* 2005; **9:** S30–S31(abstract; paper in press with PLOS).

9. Bhopal R, Fischbacher C, Vartiainen E, Unwin N, White M, Alberti G. Predicted and observed cardiovascular disease in South Asians: application of FINRISK, Framingham and SCORE models to Newcastle Heart Project data. *Journal of Public Health* 2005; **27**: 93–100.

10. Gill PS, Kai J, Bhopal RS, Wild S. Health Care Needs Assessment: Black and Minority Ethnic Groups. The epidemiologically based needs assessment reviews. Raftery J et al (eds). In press. Available at: http://hcna.radcliffe-oxford.com/bemgframe.html